Pharmacy Technician Study Guide PTCB 2024-2025

The Ultimate PTCB study guide | Ace the Pharmacy Technician Certification Board Exam on Your First Try with No Effort

Table of contents:

Introduction

Welcome to the Pharmacy Technician Study Guide PTCB 2024-2025. This comprehensive guide is designed to provide you with the knowledge, strategies, and confidence you need to successfully pass the Pharmacy Technician Certification Board (PTCB) Exam and begin your rewarding career as a Pharmacy Technician.

Becoming a certified Pharmacy Technician is a rewarding and challenging journey. It requires a deep understanding of medications, patient safety, order entry, processing, and much more. This book will guide you through each of these topics in a clear, concise manner, ensuring you are well-prepared for your exam and future career.

In Chapter 1, we will explore the path to becoming a certified Pharmacy Technician. We will delve into the prerequisites, the application process, and what to expect once you are certified. This chapter will provide you with a roadmap to your certification and beyond.

Chapter 2 is dedicated to understanding the Pharmacy Technician Certification Board (PTCB) Exam. We will break down the structure of the exam, the types of questions you can expect, and the scoring system. This chapter will demystify the exam, helping you to approach it with confidence.

In Chapter 3, we focus on the PTCE, or the Pharmacy Technician Certification Exam. This chapter will provide you with a comprehensive overview of the exam, including its format, the topics it covers, and the best strategies for success.

Chapter 4 explores the role of a Pharmacy Technician in depth. We will discuss the responsibilities and duties of a Pharmacy Technician, the skills required for the job, and the various settings in which you might work. This chapter will give you a clear picture of what to expect in your future career.

Chapter 5 delves into the world of medications. We will cover different types of medications, their uses, side effects, and contraindications. This chapter will provide you with a solid foundation in pharmacology, a crucial aspect of the Pharmacy Technician's role.

Patient safety and quality of care are at the heart of the Pharmacy Technician's role, and Chapter 6 will provide you with the knowledge you need to excel in these areas. We will discuss best practices for ensuring patient safety, maintaining quality of care, and adhering to ethical and legal standards in the pharmacy.

In Chapter 7, we will cover the critical area of order entry and processing. This chapter will equip you with the practical skills you need to accurately and efficiently process prescriptions, manage inventory, and ensure the smooth operation of the pharmacy.

Finally, in Chapter 8, we provide a full-length practice test. This test will allow you to apply everything you've learned and identify areas where you might need further study. The practice test is designed to mimic the actual PTCB exam, giving you a realistic idea of what to expect on the big day.

Chapter 1: How to Become a Certified Pharmacy Technician

If you're interested in a fulfilling job in the healthcare field, consider becoming a certified pharmacy technician. Working alongside pharmacists, pharmacy technicians ensure patients receive their prescribed medications in a timely and safe manner. Their duties extend beyond assisting pharmacists, as they also fill prescriptions, manage inventory, and interact with patients.

To become a certified pharmacy technician, you need to follow a few steps. Firstly, enroll in a pharmacy technician training program offered by community colleges or vocational schools. These programs usually take about a year to complete and cover topics such as pharmacology and medication administration, which are crucial for working in a pharmacy.

After completing your training, you must pass the Pharmacy Technician Certification Exam (PTCE). This certification, issued by the Pharmacy Technician Certification Board, is a requirement for becoming a certified pharmacy technician. The exam consists of multiple-choice questions, and you have 90 minutes to complete it.

Once you pass the PTCE and become a certified pharmacy technician, you can work in various settings, including retail pharmacies, hospitals, and nursing homes. To keep your certification valid, you must complete continuing education courses and renew your certification every two years.

In conclusion, becoming a certified pharmacy technician is an excellent entry point into the healthcare industry, allowing you to make a positive impact on patients' lives. By completing a training program and passing the PTCE, you equip yourself with the skills and knowledge necessary for this rewarding career.

Functions of a Certified Pharmacy Technician

As a certified pharmacy technician, you'll perform a variety of crucial tasks within a pharmacy. These tasks are designed to assist pharmacists in ensuring patients receive safe and effective medication management. Here are some key functions of a certified pharmacy technician:

1. Filling Prescriptions: A primary role of a pharmacy technician is to help fill prescriptions. This involves verifying patient information, counting or measuring medication, and labeling prescriptions for dispensing.

2. Managing Inventory: Pharmacy technicians are in charge of maintaining inventory levels and ensuring medications are correctly stored and labeled. This includes ordering and receiving medications, checking expiration dates, and monitoring medication stock levels.

3. Communicating with Patients: Pharmacy technicians often interact directly with patients. They answer questions about medications, explain dosage instructions, and provide general information about pharmacy services.

4. Compounding Medications: In some pharmacies, technicians may be tasked with compounding medications. This process involves mixing or preparing medications in a sterile environment.

5. Ensuring Compliance: Pharmacy technicians ensure all pharmacy operations adhere to state and federal regulations. This includes maintaining accurate records, following safety protocols, and adhering to ethical standards.

In summary, the functions of a certified pharmacy technician are vital for a pharmacy's smooth operation. By performing these tasks with accuracy and care, pharmacy technicians play a significant role in ensuring patient safety and well-being.

Career Options

Being a certified pharmacy technician opens up a wide range of career opportunities within the healthcare sector. The demand for pharmacy technicians is expected to increase in the coming years, providing ample opportunities for those seeking to enter this field. Here are some career paths that certified pharmacy technicians can consider:

1. Retail Pharmacy: This is a common career choice for pharmacy technicians, where they work in drug stores, supermarkets, and other retail environments. Their duties include filling prescriptions, managing stock, and interacting with customers.

2. Hospital Pharmacy: Pharmacy technicians can also work in hospitals, where they prepare and distribute medications to patients. They may also collaborate with other healthcare professionals to ensure patients are receiving the correct medication.

3. Long-term Care Pharmacy: Pharmacy technicians are often employed in long-term care facilities like nursing homes and assisted living centers. Here, they work alongside healthcare professionals to manage the medication plans for residents.

4. Compounding Pharmacy: In compounding pharmacies, pharmacy technicians prepare customized medications for patients with specific needs. This involves mixing, measuring, and packaging medications under the supervision of a pharmacist.

5. Specialty Pharmacy: Pharmacy technicians can also work in specialty pharmacies, helping manage medications for patients with chronic illnesses or complex medication schedules.

Each of these career paths offers unique responsibilities and opportunities for growth. By choosing a career in pharmacy, you can make a positive impact on patients' lives and contribute to the success of the healthcare industry.

Remuneration

The salary and benefits for a certified pharmacy technician are highly competitive. The compensation varies based on location, experience, and the employer. However, pharmacy technicians can expect a steady income with potential for growth.

In May 2020, the median annual wage for pharmacy technicians in the United States was $34,890, as per the Bureau of Labor Statistics. The highest earners made over $49,130 annually, while the lowest earners made less than $24,120.

Pharmacy technicians may also receive competitive salaries and benefits such as retirement plans, health insurance, and paid leave. Some employers may even offer tuition reimbursement programs to help pharmacy technicians further their education and career.

Overall, the compensation for certified pharmacy technicians reflects their vital role in the healthcare industry. Besides earning a steady income, pharmacy technicians also enjoy various benefits and have the opportunity to make a positive impact on patients' lives.

The Advantages of Being a CPhT.

Choosing to become a certified pharmacy technician (CPhT) comes with numerous benefits. These professionals play a vital role in the healthcare sector, working hand in hand with pharmacists to guarantee that patients get safe and effective medication therapy. Here are some of the advantages of becoming a CPhT:

1. Increasing Demand: The need for pharmacy technicians is on the rise, creating more opportunities for those interested in this field. This increase in demand is largely due to an aging population that necessitates more healthcare services.

2. Career Progression: Being a CPhT can open doors for career progression. With further education and training, pharmacy technicians can specialize in areas like compounding, sterile product preparation, and medication therapy management.

3. Attractive Salary: Pharmacy technicians can expect a competitive salary with the possibility of growth over time. In addition to a steady income, health insurance and retirement plans may be offered to pharmacy technicians.

4. Work Flexibility: Pharmacy technicians have the advantage of a flexible work schedule, with numerous options for both part-time and

full-time employment. This flexibility can be particularly beneficial for those with other responsibilities, such as family or education.

5. Rewarding Work: Most importantly, being a CPhT allows you to positively impact the lives of patients in your community. As a pharmacy technician, you can work directly with patients, ensuring they receive safe and effective medication therapy.

Choosing to become a certified pharmacy technician can offer many rewards, from career progression to fulfilling work. By choosing a career in pharmacy, you'll have the chance to contribute to the overall success of the healthcare industry while enjoying a stable and rewarding career.

Chapter 2: Understanding the Pharmacy Technician Certification Board (PTCB) Exam

The Importance of PTCB Certification

The PTCB certification is of great value to those who wish to pursue a career as pharmacy technicians. It serves as a testament to their skills, knowledge, and proficiency in this field. As the healthcare landscape continues to evolve, pharmacy technicians play a crucial role in maintaining patient safety and delivering quality care. Hence, acquiring a PTCB certification is an essential step in establishing oneself as a competent professional in the pharmacy sector.

Acquiring a PTCB certification is a testament to one's dedication to excellence and professionalism. It indicates that a pharmacy technician has met the stringent standards set by the PTCB, a recognized authority in the field. The certification process evaluates a broad spectrum of knowledge areas, including pharmacy calculations, medication safety, pharmacy law, inventory management, and more. Passing the exam successfully showcases a comprehensive understanding of these vital topics.

A PTCB certification can open up a range of career opportunities in the pharmacy industry. Many employers now prefer or require candidates to have a PTCB certification, as it assures them of the technician's proficiency and commitment to the profession. The certification serves as proof of one's dedication to maintaining high practice standards and staying abreast of the latest advancements in the field.

Furthermore, obtaining a PTCB certification brings a sense of personal achievement and pride. It signifies the culmination of hours of study, preparation, and hard work. For pharmacy technicians, it is a significant milestone that underscores their dedication to professional development and progression. A PTCB certification serves as a motivation to continually enhance skills and stay updated with industry changes.

Besides personal and professional benefits, a PTCB certification also contributes to patient safety. Pharmacy technicians, as medication experts, play a vital role in ensuring accurate medication dispensing, preventing errors, and promoting medication adherence. By maintaining their certification, technicians show their commitment to upholding the highest safety and quality standards in medication management. Patients can trust that certified pharmacy technicians have the knowledge and skills to assist in their healthcare journey.

The PTCB certification is recognized and respected across the country. It provides a standardized measure for evaluating the competence of pharmacy technicians. By adhering to strict standards and offering a comprehensive examination process, the PTCB ensures that certified technicians can meet the demands of the ever-changing healthcare industry.

Acquiring a PTCB certification is a significant achievement for pharmacy technicians. It showcases their proficiency, professionalism, and dedication to patient safety. The certification paves the way for new career opportunities, enhances personal and professional growth, and contributes to the overall quality of healthcare. Aspiring pharmacy technicians should consider PTCB certification as a critical step in their journey towards a successful and rewarding career in the pharmacy field.

Overview of the PTCB Exam

The Pharmacy Technician Certification Board (PTCB) exam is a thorough evaluation designed to measure the knowledge and skills of prospective pharmacy technicians. This exam is pivotal in gauging the proficiency of candidates and their capability to execute tasks vital to the pharmacy profession. By passing the PTCB exam, individuals prove their preparedness to join the field and contribute to the provision of safe and efficient patient care.

The PTCB exam encompasses a broad spectrum of topics pertinent to pharmacy practice. It gauges candidates' comprehension of pharmaceutical calculations, drug classifications and terminology, pharmacy law and regulations, medication order entry and processing, medication safety and quality assurance, pharmacy information systems, medication adherence and patient education, and compounding and sterile preparations. The exam is designed to evaluate both theoretical knowledge and practical skills necessary for pharmacy technicians to thrive in their roles.

The PTCB exam is composed of multiple-choice questions (MCQs), requiring candidates to choose the most suitable answer from a list of options. These questions are meticulously designed to assess the depth and breadth of candidates' understanding in various pharmacy-related fields. The exam may also include situational questions that evaluate candidates' capability to apply their knowledge in real-life situations.

To ensure the exam's fairness and validity, the PTCB adheres to strict standards in test development. The exam content is regularly reviewed and updated to keep pace with the changing demands of the pharmacy profession. Experts in the subject matter, including active pharmacy technicians and pharmacists, contribute to the creation and validation of exam questions to ensure their relevance and accuracy.

Thorough preparation for the PTCB exam is crucial for candidates to maximize their chances of success. This might involve studying comprehensive textbooks, attending review courses, using online resources, and practicing with sample questions and mock exams. Becoming familiar with the exam format, content areas, and time management strategies can significantly improve overall performance.

Achieving PTCB certification by passing the exam is a notable accomplishment for pharmacy technicians. It signifies their commitment to professional development, adherence to industry standards, and dedication to delivering optimal patient care. PTCB certification is widely acknowledged and respected in the pharmacy field, paving the way for various job opportunities and career progression.

The PTCB exam acts as a stringent assessment of the knowledge and skills necessary to be a proficient pharmacy technician. It covers a wide array of pharmacy-related topics and evaluates candidates' abilities to apply their knowledge in practical situations. By successfully passing the exam, individuals prove their readiness to contribute to the pharmacy profession and ensure the safe and effective use of medications.

Chapter 3: The PTCE

Eligibility Criteria

To qualify for the PTCE, certain prerequisites must be met. These are as follows:

1. High School Degree or Equivalent: You must possess a high school diploma or its equivalent, such as a GED, to be eligible for the test. If you are a high school student nearing graduation (within 60 days), you may be allowed to take the test.

2. No Criminal Record: You must not have any felony or drug- or pharmacy-related convictions.

3. No Drug or Pharmacy-related Board of Pharmacy Sanctions: You must not have any restrictions, suspensions, revocations, or other actions from the Board of Pharmacy related to drug or pharmacy-related activities.

4. Adherence to PTCB Certification Policies: You must abide by all PTCB certification policies, which include the Continuing Education Policy, the Code of Conduct, and the PTCB Certification Program Policies.

5. Compliance with State and Federal Laws: You must adhere to all state and federal laws associated with pharmacy practice.

Remember that eligibility criteria might differ from state to state. Therefore, you should consult your state's Board of Pharmacy to confirm you meet all the prerequisites before registering for the test. Additionally, fulfilling the eligibility criteria does not assure a pass in the test. Adequate preparation is crucial to enhance your chances of success.

Procedure to Register for the Exam

Before registering for the PTCE, you need to create an account on the PTCB website. Once your account is set up, follow the steps below to register for the test:

1. Confirm Your Eligibility: Prior to registering for the PTCE, make sure you fulfill all the eligibility criteria. This includes having a high school degree or equivalent, no criminal record or drug-related offenses, and no violations of PTCB certification rules.

2. Select an Exam Date and Venue: After confirming your eligibility, choose a suitable exam date and location. The PTCE is conducted at Pearson VUE test centers throughout the United States. You can look up available test centers and dates on the PTCB website.

3. Pay the Exam Fee: The PTCE costs $149. You can pay this fee online using a credit or debit card. If you need financial aid to pay for the test, you may qualify for the PTCB's Exam Assistance Program.

4. Schedule Your Exam: Once you've paid the fee, you can book your exam slot at a Pearson VUE test center. You will receive a confirmation email with your exam appointment details.

5. Prepare for the Exam: Thorough preparation is crucial to pass the PTCE. The PTCB provides several study resources, such as a Candidate Guide, a Content Outline, and practice tests. Additionally, you can find various study guides and test prep books in the market that could be beneficial.

Remember that you can register and take the PTCE at any time as registration is open all year round. However, it's advisable to register early to secure your preferred exam date and location.

Setting Up an Exam

The process of setting up your exam is a crucial part of the certification process. After fulfilling all the necessary prerequisites and registering for the exam, it's time to set up your test appointment.

Firstly, look over the testing options available to you and select a date and location that is most convenient. You have the option to set up your exam either online or over the phone. Keep in mind that testing centers have limited space, so it's advisable to set up your appointment as early as possible to secure your preferred date and time.

Ensure to arrive at the testing location at least 30 minutes prior to your scheduled appointment to complete any required check-in procedures. The testing center may require additional documents, so make sure to bring these along with your two forms of ID.

Take note that if you need to reschedule or cancel your exam, you may be charged additional fees, so plan accordingly and be ready for your exam day. Good luck!

Changing/Canceling the Exam

If you need to change or cancel your PTCE exam, it's crucial to do so in a timely and proper manner. You must make these changes at least 48 hours before the scheduled exam time. If you don't, you'll lose your exam fee and will have to pay the fee again to set up another exam.

To change or cancel your exam, you need to get in touch with Pearson VUE, the company that oversees the PTCE exam. You can either call them or visit their website to make the request. Remember that if you reschedule your exam, you may not get your preferred testing location or date as these slots are filled quickly.

Please note that you can only change or cancel your exam up to two times. After that, you'll need to submit a new application and pay the exam fee again. Therefore, it's advisable to only change or cancel your exam if absolutely necessary.

In summary, if you need to change or cancel your PTCE exam, contact Pearson VUE directly at least 48 hours before the scheduled exam time, and remember that you can only change or cancel up to two times.

No-Show Policy

The P.T.C.B. has a no-show policy in place to ensure the efficient use of testing centers and to provide all test-takers with equal opportunities to schedule exams. If you miss your scheduled exam appointment, you will lose your fee and will have to pay the full fee to reschedule.

To avoid losing your exam fee, it's crucial to carefully schedule your exam appointment and make sure that you can attend on the specified date and time. If for any reason you cannot make your scheduled appointment, make sure to change or cancel in advance to avoid additional fees or penalties.

It's important to note that the no-show policy also applies to candidates who arrive more than 15 minutes late for their scheduled exam appointment. If you're running late, it's best to contact the testing center as soon as possible to discuss your options and avoid losing your exam fee.

By being aware of the P.T.C.B.'s no-show policy and avoiding missing or being late for your exam appointment, you can ensure a successful and stress-free testing experience.

Retake Policies

If you don't succeed in passing the PTCE on your initial try, you'll have the opportunity to retake it after a 60-day waiting period. You're allowed to take the PTCE up to four times within a year, with a six-month waiting period required between the fourth and fifth attempts.

Keep in mind that there's a fee for each retake. If you don't pass the PTCE on your first go, you'll have to pay the full exam fee for a second attempt. For any subsequent attempts, the fee will be reduced.

To improve your chances of passing the PTCE on your next try, it's recommended you review your exam score report to identify the areas where you performed poorly. Concentrate your studies on these areas and consider using additional resources like review courses or study guides.

Remember, some states may have extra requirements for retaking the PTCE. Make sure to check with your state's pharmacy board to ensure you meet all necessary requirements.

Recertification

Certified Pharmacy Technicians (CPhTs) are required to renew their certification every two years to maintain their professional status. If you don't renew your certification within this period, it will expire.

To recertify as a CPhT, you're required to complete 20 hours of Continuing Education (CE) during each certification cycle. The Pharmacy Technician Certification Board (PTCB) must approve these hours. At least two hours should be dedicated to patient safety, and one hour should focus on pharmacy legislation.

Besides completing the necessary CE hours, CPhTs must apply for recertification and pay a recertification fee. The application must be submitted online via the PTCB website, with the fee paid at the time of submission.

CPhTs should start planning for recertification as soon as they get certified to ensure they have ample time to complete the required CE hours and submit their application. Failure to recertify by the deadline will result in loss of certification, and you'll need to retake the PTCE to regain your certification.

Staying certified as a CPhT is crucial for maintaining your knowledge and skills as a pharmacy technician. By keeping up with the latest advancements in pharmacy, CPhTs can provide the best care to patients and contribute positively to their workplace.

What to Expect on the Exam Day

Feeling nervous on the day of your PTCE is common, but being aware of what to expect can help reduce your anxiety. Here's what you need to know about the exam day:

1. Arrival time: It's advised to arrive at the testing site 30 minutes before the exam begins. This will give you enough time to check in, store your belongings, and fill out the necessary paperwork.

2. Required items: You'll need to bring two forms of ID, one of which should be a government-issued photo ID like a driver's license or passport. Also, remember to bring a printout of your exam registration confirmation.

3. What you can bring: You're allowed to bring a basic calculator, a noticeboard or whiteboard, and a dry-erase marker for the exam. If you think the testing center might be chilly, you can also bring a jacket or sweater.

4. What you can't bring: Personal items like cell phones, food, or drinks are not allowed in the testing room. Study materials or notes are also prohibited.

5. Exam format: The PTCE consists of 90 multiple-choice questions that you'll need to answer within two hours. The questions don't follow a specific order, so make sure to read each one thoroughly before answering.

6. Computer-based testing: The PTCE is a computer-based test, so basic computer skills like using a mouse and keyboard are necessary. There's also an optional tutorial at the start of the exam to help you get acquainted with the testing software.

7. Breaks: You're allowed a 10-minute break during the exam, but this will be deducted from your total testing time.

Being aware of what to expect on your PTCE day can help reduce your anxiety and prepare you better for success.

Exam Delivery Methods

The Pharmacy Technician Certification Exam (PTCE) can be taken in two ways: through computer-based testing (CBT) or remote proctoring (RP). Unlike RP, which requires you to be at a Pearson VUE testing center, CBT allows you to take the test from the comfort of your home or office.

Computer-Based Testing (CBT)

With CBT, you can take the PTCE at a nearby Pearson VUE testing center. A computer will be provided for you to take the test, and you'll receive your results immediately afterwards. CBT exams are held at various times and locations throughout the year, giving you the flexibility to choose a date and location that suits you best.

Remote Proctoring (RP)

RP allows you to take the PTCE from any location, as long as you have an internet connection. You'll need a computer equipped with a webcam and microphone, as well as a quiet, private space to take the test. An online proctor will supervise you during the test to ensure its security and prevent any cheating. RP provides the convenience of taking the test from your chosen location, without the need to travel to a testing center.

Please note that both CBT and RP require strict adherence to rules and procedures to maintain the exam's integrity. Make sure to review the policies and procedures for the delivery method you choose before scheduling your exam.

Regulations and Rules

As a PTCE candidate, it's crucial to familiarize yourself with the rules and regulations set by the Pharmacy Technician Certification Board (PTCB). These rules are in place to safeguard the exam's validity and the overall credibility of the certification process.

Here are some key rules and regulations to remember:

1. Identification: You'll need to present a government-issued photo ID and another form of identification with your name at the testing center.

2. Check-in process: Upon arrival at the testing center, you'll go through a check-in process that includes having your photo taken, verifying your ID, and storing your personal items in a locker.

3. Test duration: The PTCE consists of 90 multiple-choice questions and lasts for two hours.

4. Breaks: You're allowed to take breaks during the test, but the timer will keep running. You're not permitted to access your personal items during the break.

5. Test content: The exam primarily covers four topics: Federal Requirements (12.5%), Medications (40%), Patient Safety and Order Entry and Processing (6.25%), and Quality Assurance (26.25%).

6. Banned items: No external items, including but not limited to food, drinks, or study aids, are allowed in the testing room.

7. Cheating: Cheating is strictly forbidden and will lead to immediate disqualification from the test.

8. Test results: Your test results will be available within two to three weeks after the test date. If you pass, you'll receive a certificate and can use the CPhT designation.

By adhering to these rules and regulations, you can ensure a smooth testing experience and increase your chances of passing the PTCE and obtaining your certification.

Explaining the Exam Development Process

The Pharmacy Technician Certification Exam (PTCE), created by the Pharmacy Technician Certification Board (PTCB), is a requirement for those aspiring to be certified pharmacy technicians. The PTCB, an independent, non-profit organization, is responsible for the certification of pharmacy technicians across the United States.

The PTCE is meticulously developed through a process that involves subject matter experts (SMEs), including experienced pharmacists and pharmacy technicians from various pharmacy settings, as well as psychometricians, who specialize in test development and assessment.

A job analysis study, conducted every five years, forms the basis of the PTCE. This study ensures that the exam remains relevant and up-to-date with current pharmacy practices. Researchers survey thousands of technicians working in retail, institutional, and compounding pharmacies to determine the necessary education and experience for effective performance in their roles.

The findings from the job analysis study guide the SMEs in creating a comprehensive content outline for the PTCE. This outline details the topics and subtopics to be covered in the exam, and the proportion of questions dedicated to each topic.

The SMEs then create test items or questions, which are reviewed and edited by experts for precision and clarity. A group of pharmacy technicians pretests these items to validate their reliability.

Once the items are finalized, they are compiled into various versions of the PTCE, and equated to ensure equal difficulty across all versions. Equating is a method that compares the difficulty levels of different exam versions and adjusts the scores accordingly, ensuring fair scoring for all test takers, regardless of the exam version they take.

In essence, the development of the PTCE is a comprehensive and meticulous process that ensures the exam is valid, reliable, and fair for all test takers. Understanding this process can help pharmacy technicians feel confident that the PTCE accurately assesses their pharmacy knowledge and skills.

Understanding Exam Scoring

The PTCE is scored on a 1,000-point scale, with a passing score being 650 or above. This means you need to answer at least 65% of the questions correctly to pass. The scoring is done using a computerized adaptive testing (CAT) system, which adjusts the difficulty of the questions based on your performance.

Each question on the exam carries one point, and there's no penalty for guessing. Therefore, it's advisable to answer all questions, even if you're unsure.

The PTCE tests various areas, including medication safety, pharmacy legislation and regulations, order entry and fill procedure, prescription information, and pharmacy calculations.

Your final score is determined by the number of correct answers and the difficulty level of those questions. If you answer a question correctly, the computer presents a more challenging question. If your answer is incorrect, the system presents a simpler question.

It's important to note that the PTCE is a pass/fail exam, so you won't receive a numerical score. Your test performance will be communicated to you in text form. If you don't pass on your first attempt, you can retake the exam after a 60-day waiting period.

In conclusion, the PTCE is scored on a 1,000-point scale, with a passing score of 650 or higher. The scoring is done using a computerized adaptive testing system, which adjusts the difficulty of the questions based on your performance. To pass, you need to answer at least 65% of the questions correctly.

Receiving PTCE Results

After taking the PTCE, you might be curious about when and how you'll get your results. Fortunately, you won't have to wait too long because the computer-based exam is scored instantly once you finish it.

Shortly after the test, your preliminary scores will be handed to you. You'll discover whether you've passed or failed, and you'll also get a scaled score ranging from 1,000 to 1,600. To pass the PTCE, you need a score of 1,400 or more, so it's important to strive for this score.

Keep in mind that the information you gather now is not final. The PTCE is a computer-adaptive test, meaning the complexity of the questions you receive adjusts based on your performance on previous questions. As a result, your projected grades may slightly vary after a more detailed examination of your test has been conducted.

Official score reports are usually available one to three weeks after the test date. You can find your official score report in your PTCB account. If you pass the exam, a certificate will be sent to you within two to four weeks from the score report's release date.

If you don't pass the PTCE on your first try, you can retake it after a 60-day period from the initial exam date. It's crucial to review your score report before retaking the test to identify what you've mastered and what you still need to learn.

In summary, you'll be able to see your unofficial results immediately after the test, and your official score report will be accessible within one to three weeks. If you don't pass on your first attempt, you can retake the test after 60 days. If you pass, a certificate will be mailed to you.

Guidance for Passing the Exam

Preparing for the PTCE can seem overwhelming, but there are measures you can take to enhance your likelihood of passing. Here are some suggestions for your preparation:

1. Consistent and regular study: The key to acing the PTCE is to study consistently and regularly. Create a study plan and stick to it, dedicating sufficient time each day or week to go over all the essential topics.

2. Understand the exam content: Get acquainted with the exam content by going through the PTCE Content Outline. Ensure you comprehend the knowledge areas and topics that will be tested.

3. Practice with sample questions: Utilize study guides and practice tests that provide sample questions. Practicing with a variety of questions will help you get comfortable with the exam's format and content.

4. Concentrate on your weak areas: Identify and focus your study efforts on these areas. Use the PTCE Content Outline to help you pinpoint the areas where you need the most improvement.

5. Take care of yourself: In the weeks leading up to the exam, ensure you're taking care of your physical and mental health. Get enough sleep, eat healthily, and take breaks when necessary. Being well-rested and rejuvenated on exam day can help you stay focused and alert.

6. Follow instructions carefully: Make sure to read and follow all exam instructions, including marking your answer sheet and taking breaks. This can help you avoid careless errors and increase your chances of success.

7. Stay calm and confident: Lastly, maintain your calm and confidence on exam day. Remember that you've prepared well and are ready for the exam. Take a deep breath, read each question carefully, and concentrate on answering to the best of your ability.

By adhering to these tips and investing the necessary time and effort in preparation, you can boost your chances of passing the PTCE and earning your pharmacy technician certification.

How to Study

Effective preparation for the PTCB exam involves strategic planning and readiness. Here are some suggestions to optimize your study time:

1. Create a study strategy: Prior to diving into your studies, design a plan detailing what you need to study and the time you'll dedicate to it. Segment the material into digestible parts and establish a feasible timetable for yourself. This strategy will keep you focused and guarantee that you go through all the necessary content before the day of the exam.

2. Utilize various study tools: To better comprehend the material, use a variety of study aids. These can include textbooks, online materials, flashcards, mock exams, and study groups. Each tool provides unique perspectives and aids in consolidating what you've learned.

3. Concentrate on key subjects: Although it's crucial to cover all the material, certain subjects may carry more weight in the exam than others. Pay special attention to drug classifications, dosage computations, and pharmacy law to ensure you have a thorough understanding of these topics.

4. Constant practice: Practice questions are crucial for PTCB exam preparation. They not only enhance your understanding of the material but also familiarize you with the exam structure and test-taking techniques. Practice exams can also help pinpoint areas where you need to concentrate more.

5. Incorporate breaks: Studying for extended periods can be exhausting, hence the need for recharging. Incorporate short breaks every hour or so, and take longer breaks when required. Engage in

physical activity, go for a walk, or do something relaxing to refresh your mind and alleviate stress.

By adhering to these guidelines, you can create an effective study strategy and set yourself up for success in the PTCB exam.

Chapter 4: The Role of a Pharmacy Technician

Examining the Duties and Practice Boundaries

A pharmacy technician's primary duty is to aid pharmacists in the distribution of medicines. They handle and process prescriptions, ensuring they are accurate and complete. This includes confirming patient details, scrutinizing the prescription for potential drug interactions or contraindications, and choosing the correct medications. Pharmacy technicians are also crucial in the labeling and packaging of medicines, ensuring they are properly prepared for distribution to patients.

Aside from dispensing medicines, pharmacy technicians are tasked with keeping precise patient records and medication profiles. They input and update patient data in the pharmacy information system, safeguarding the privacy and accuracy of patient information. This data is vital for tracking medication usage, spotting potential drug interactions, and delivering comprehensive pharmaceutical care.

Pharmacy technicians also assist with inventory management in the pharmacy. They help in the acquisition, storage, and organization of medicines and supplies. This involves monitoring medication inventory levels, inspecting for expired or damaged items, and ensuring correct storage conditions. Through maintaining an effective inventory system, pharmacy technicians aid in preventing medication shortages and guaranteeing the availability of necessary medicines to patients.

Providing excellent customer service is another key aspect of a pharmacy technician's role. They engage with patients, answering their queries and providing information related to medications. This can include explaining medication directions, discussing potential side effects, and offering advice on correct medication usage. Effective communication skills and a caring approach are essential in establishing trust with patients and ensuring their understanding of their medications.

Understanding the boundaries and scope of their practice is vital for pharmacy technicians. While they work closely with pharmacists, certain tasks are exclusively the responsibility of the pharmacist. Pharmacy technicians must adhere to legal and ethical rules and avoid performing tasks that go beyond their authorized practice boundaries. This ensures patient safety and compliance with regulatory standards.

Pharmacy technicians are a crucial part of the healthcare team, collaborating with pharmacists and other healthcare professionals to provide optimal patient care. Their role goes beyond dispensing medication and includes various duties related to patient safety, inventory management, and customer service. By diligently fulfilling their duties within their authorized practice boundaries, pharmacy technicians enhance the overall efficiency and effectiveness of the pharmacy setting.

In conclusion, pharmacy technicians are vital in supporting pharmacists and ensuring the safe and efficient provision of medications to patients. Their duties encompass medication dispensing, record maintenance, inventory management, and patient education. By understanding their practice boundaries and diligently performing their duties, pharmacy technicians significantly contribute to the delivery of quality pharmaceutical care.

Understanding the Impact of Pharmacy Technicians in Healthcare

Pharmacy technicians play a substantial role in the healthcare sector, enhancing the quality of patient care. Their pivotal roles and duties support the smooth operations of pharmacies and enhance the management of medications. It's essential to acknowledge the influence of pharmacy technicians in healthcare to appreciate the value they add to the healthcare team.

A significant contribution of pharmacy technicians is their involvement in medication safety. They are fundamental in ensuring that drugs are dispensed correctly, in compliance with the set protocols and guidelines. Pharmacy technicians aid in reducing medication mistakes by rechecking prescriptions, confirming patient details, and comparing medication orders with patient profiles. Their meticulousness and adherence to best practices enhance patient safety and lower the likelihood of adverse drug incidents.

Pharmacy technicians also help in encouraging patients to stick to their medication regimen. They actively participate in educating patients, offering information about drugs, their functions, correct usage, and possible side effects. By providing clear directions and addressing patient queries, pharmacy technicians enable patients to follow their medication prescriptions, resulting in better health results and disease control.

Besides their direct patient interactions, pharmacy technicians aid the healthcare team by handling administrative duties. They assist in keeping precise records of drug dispensing, oversee medication stock, and facilitate communication between healthcare providers and patients. Pharmacy technicians are skilled in using pharmacy information systems, which simplify documentation procedures, boost communication, and enhance overall efficiency in managing medications.

Pharmacy technicians are also crucial in enhancing healthcare accessibility and affordability. With their expertise, they aid in executing medication assistance schemes, like patient assistance programs and medication discount cards. By assisting patients in navigating these programs, pharmacy technicians ensure that individuals can access the medications they require, irrespective of their financial situation. This dedication to patient advocacy encourages equal healthcare access and improves patient outcomes.

Moreover, pharmacy technicians boost the overall efficiency of the healthcare system. By effectively managing medication stock, they help avoid medication shortages and ensure the availability of necessary drugs. They aid in optimizing drug use and reducing waste, resulting in cost savings for healthcare organizations. Their role in simplifying processes and maintaining an organized pharmacy environment contributes to efficient healthcare service delivery.

Pharmacy technicians are essential members of the healthcare team, offering valuable support to pharmacists, healthcare professionals, and patients. Their impact goes beyond the pharmacy, reaching patients in different healthcare environments. With their expertise, abilities, and commitment to patient care, pharmacy technicians contribute to enhanced medication safety, improved patient education, increased healthcare access, and overall healthcare system efficiency.

Chapter 5: Medications

Pharmaceutical Classifications, Naming Conventions, and Brand Names

Understanding the various names and categories of drugs is crucial for a pharmacy technician. Each medication has a generic name, which is the name of the active ingredient, and it's typically cheaper than the brand-name versions. The brand name, however, is the name given by the manufacturer and is often more well-known to patients.

Drugs are also categorized based on their therapeutic uses or how they work. Here are some common drug classifications:

- Analgesics: These are pain-relieving drugs like acetaminophen, ibuprofen, and oxycodone.

- Antacids: These neutralize stomach acids and include calcium carbonate and magnesium hydroxide.

- Antibiotics: These treat bacterial infections and include amoxicillin, azithromycin, and ciprofloxacin.

- Anticoagulants: These prevent blood clots and include warfarin and heparin.

- Antidepressants: These treat depression and other mood disorders and include fluoxetine, sertraline, and bupropion.

- Antihypertensives: These lower blood pressure and include lisinopril, amlodipine, and metoprolol.

- Antipsychotics: These treat schizophrenia and other psychotic disorders and include risperidone, quetiapine, and olanzapine.

- Diuretics: These increase urine output and include furosemide, hydrochlorothiazide, and spironolactone.
- Estrogens: These hormones are involved in the development and maintenance of female reproductive tissues and secondary sexual characteristics.
- Erythropoiesis-stimulating agents (ESAs): These stimulate red blood cell production to treat anemia.
- Expectorants: These thin and loosen mucus in the respiratory tract to make coughing easier and more productive.
- Eye lubricants: These are used to lubricate the eyes and relieve dryness or irritation.
- Fibrates: These treat high cholesterol and triglyceride levels.
- Fluoroquinolones: These are antibiotics used to treat bacterial infections.
- Folate antagonists: These block the action of folic acid, necessary for cell growth and division, and are used to treat cancer, rheumatoid arthritis, and psoriasis.
- Fungal infections: These are treatments for fungal infections such as athlete's foot, ringworm, and thrush. Some common ones are nystatin, fluconazole, and itraconazole.
- Furosemide: This is a type of loop diuretic prescribed for patients with hypertension and fluid retention.
- Glucocorticoids: These treat inflammation and autoimmune disorders such as rheumatoid arthritis and asthma.
- Gastrointestinal agents: These treat various conditions related to the digestive system, such as acid reflux and irritable bowel syndrome.

- Gonadotropin-releasing hormone (GnRH) agonists: These are used in the treatment of breast cancer, prostate cancer, and endometriosis.

- GABA analogs: These act on the neurotransmitter gamma-aminobutyric acid and are used to treat anxiety disorders and epilepsy.

- Glycemic control agents: These are diabetic blood sugar-regulating drugs, such as insulin and metformin.

- Gamma-aminobutyric acid (GABA) receptor modulators: These are used to treat anxiety, insomnia, and seizures.

- Gallstone solubilizing agents: These dissolve gallstones and are often used when surgery is not an option.

- Glaucoma agents: These treat elevated intraocular pressure, which can cause permanent vision loss if unchecked.

- Gout agents: These are prescribed for the treatment of gout, a form of arthritis brought on by an accumulation of uric acid in the joints.

- Gonadotropins: These are hormones that stimulate the ovaries or testes to produce eggs or sperm and are used in fertility treatments.

- Hypoglycemics: These are diabetic blood sugar-lowering drugs, including metformin, insulin, and glipizide.

- H1 Antihistamines: These block the action of histamine, a chemical in the body that causes allergic reactions. Examples include diphenhydramine (Benadryl) and loratadine (Claritin).

- H2 Antagonists: These prevent histamine from stimulating acid-producing cells in the stomach, hence reducing stomach acid production. Ranitidine (Zantac) and famotidine are two such medications (Pepcid).

- Hematopoietic Agents: These stimulate the production of blood cells. Examples include erythropoietin (Epogen) and filgrastim (Neupogen).
- Hormones: These mimic the action of hormones in the body. Examples include insulin (used to treat diabetes), estrogen (used in hormone replacement therapy), and testosterone (used to treat hypogonadism).
- Hypnotics: These promote sleep. Examples include zolpidem (Ambien) and temazepam (Restoril).
- HMG-CoA Reductase Inhibitors: These lower cholesterol levels by blocking the action of an enzyme in the liver that produces cholesterol. Examples include atorvastatin (Lipitor) and simvastatin (Zocor).

It's important to realize that some drugs may fall into multiple categories based on their therapeutic uses and how they work. As a pharmacy technician, understanding the different names and categories of drugs is crucial to help patients and healthcare professionals manage their medications effectively.

Therapeutic Equivalence

The Food and Drug Administration (FDA) in the United States has established guidelines to confirm that generic drugs are as safe, effective, and of the same quality as their branded equivalents. This concept is known as therapeutic equivalence.

Therapeutic equivalence involves comparing different drugs with similar active ingredients and purposes to ascertain if they produce the same therapeutic results. In essence, it signifies that two distinct drugs can be used interchangeably to achieve the same therapeutic effect.

The FDA uses a rating system in the United States to establish therapeutic equivalence. Generic drugs that have been given an "A" rating are deemed therapeutically equivalent to their branded counterparts, while those with a "B" rating are not.

It's crucial to understand that therapeutic equivalence doesn't imply that the two drugs are identical in terms of their inactive ingredients, dosage forms, or other aspects. However, it does mean that the drugs are considered equivalent in terms of their active ingredients and overall therapeutic effect.

Pharmacy technicians play a vital role in ensuring that patients are given the correct drugs, whether branded or generic. By understanding therapeutic equivalence and identifying which drugs are deemed therapeutically equivalent, pharmacy technicians can help ensure that patients receive safe, effective, and affordable medications.

Common and Potentially Fatal Drug Interactions

It's critical to consider potential drug interactions and contraindications before administering medications to patients. Here are some examples of common and potentially lethal drug interactions and contraindications:

Drug-disease interactions: Certain drugs can worsen existing health conditions or interact with a patient's medical history. For instance, patients with liver disease should avoid drugs that are metabolized in the liver, as they can exacerbate the disease.

Drug-drug interactions: Two or more drugs can interact negatively, causing adverse reactions or diminishing effectiveness. For instance, taking aspirin with a blood thinner like warfarin can increase the risk of severe bleeding complications.

Drug-dietary supplement interactions: Dietary supplements can interact with drugs, altering their effects or causing adverse reactions.

For instance, the effectiveness of some antidepressants may be reduced by St. John's wort.

Drug-laboratory interactions: Some drugs can interfere with laboratory tests, resulting in inaccurate results. For instance, steroids can alter blood glucose levels and interfere with diabetes testing.

Drug-nutrient interactions: Some drugs can affect the absorption or metabolism of nutrients, leading to nutritional deficiencies. For instance, certain antibiotics can interfere with the absorption of vitamin K, which is crucial for blood clotting.

Pharmacy technicians should be aware of these interactions and contraindications and relay this information to patients and healthcare providers to ensure the safe and effective use of medications.

Strength/Dose, Dosage Forms, Administration Routes, Special Handling and Administration Instructions, and Treatment Duration

Strength/Dose: This term refers to the quantity of the active substance present in each unit of a drug. For instance, if a prescription reads "ibuprofen 400mg tablets," it means each tablet contains 400mg of the active substance.

Dosage Forms: Medicines can come in various forms such as liquids, creams, tablets, capsules, and injections. The form of the drug can influence its absorption rate and effectiveness in the body.

Routes of Administration: This term describes how a drug is introduced into the body. Common methods include oral (through the mouth), topical (applied on the skin), inhalation (breathed in), and injection (injected into a muscle or vein).

Special Handling and Administration Instructions: Certain medications require specific handling or administration instructions to ensure they are safe and effective. For instance, insulin needs to be refrigerated and injected at the correct time and place.

Duration of Drug Therapy: This term refers to the length of time a drug should be taken or used. Some drugs are used for a short duration, like antibiotics for a week, while others are used for longer periods, such as drugs for chronic illnesses like hypertension or diabetes.

Pharmacy technicians must be well-versed in these aspects of medications to ensure patients use them safely and effectively.

Extreme and Frequent Drug Reactions

Medications can save lives, but they can also have side effects, adverse effects, and trigger allergic reactions. Pharmacy technicians need to be aware of these potential risks to help patients understand what to expect from their medication and when to seek medical help.

Common Medication Side Effects:

Patients may experience several common side effects from medications, such as:

- Nausea and vomiting
- Dizziness or lightheadedness
- Headache
- Fatigue or drowsiness
- Insomnia
- Diarrhea or constipation
- Dry mouth
- Rash or itching

If patients experience any persistent or severe side effects, they should report them to their healthcare provider as it may indicate a need for a medication or dosage adjustment.

Dangerous and Unwanted Reactions to Drugs:

Some medication side effects can be severe or even life-threatening. Severe medication side effects and adverse effects include:

- Anaphylaxis: a severe allergic reaction causing difficulty in breathing, swelling, and hives

- Stevens-Johnson Syndrome: a rare, severe skin disorder causing a painful rash and blisters
- Blood disorders: some drugs can affect blood cell counts, leading to anemia or bleeding disorders
- Liver or kidney damage: certain drugs can cause damage to these organs over time

Pharmacy technicians should be aware of these severe and adverse side effects to help patients recognize symptoms and seek medical help promptly.

Medication Allergies:

Some patients may have allergic reactions to medications. Common symptoms of medication allergies include:

- Difficulty breathing
- Hives or rash
- Face, lip, or tongue swelling
- Rapid heartbeat
- Dizziness or fainting

If a patient experience any of these symptoms after taking a medication, they should seek immediate medical attention.

Pharmacy technicians can help prevent medication allergies by reviewing patients' medical histories and checking for any known allergies before dispensing medication. They can also provide information on recognizing and responding to allergic reactions.

Drug Stability

The term "drug stability" pertains to the ability of a medication to retain its strength and efficacy over a certain period. This concept is crucial for pharmacy technicians, especially when dealing with oral suspensions, insulin, reconstitutes, injectable drugs, and vaccines.

Oral Suspensions

Oral suspensions are liquid medications with minute particles of the active substance dispersed in a liquid medium. Compared to tablets or capsules, these medications are typically less stable as the particles can settle over time, causing inconsistencies in strength. To maintain the stability of oral suspensions, pharmacy technicians are advised to:

- Store them in a cool, dry environment
- Shake the bottle thoroughly prior to use
- Dispose of any medication that is not used by the expiration date

Insulin

Insulin is a common medication used in the treatment of diabetes. It comes in various forms such as fast-acting, short-acting, intermediate-acting, and extended-release. Insulin remains stable at room temperature for up to 28 days, but for longer periods, it should be refrigerated. Pharmacy technicians should:

- Keep insulin in a refrigerator
- Verify the expiration date before dispensing
- Throw away any insulin left unused after the expiration date

Reconstitutes

Certain medications like antibiotics are provided in a powdered form that needs to be mixed with a liquid before administration. These medications are usually less stable than pre-mixed ones as the active ingredient might degrade or lose its potency when exposed to moisture or heat. To maintain the stability of reconstitutes, pharmacy technicians should:

- Adhere to the manufacturer's instructions for reconstitution
- Use the medication within the suggested time frame
- Refrigerate reconstituted medications if necessary

Injectables

Injectable medications, such as vaccines and antibiotics, require careful preparation and administration to ensure their stability and effectiveness. Pharmacy technicians should:

- Follow sterile compounding procedures when preparing injectables
- Confirm the expiration date before dispensing
- Refrigerate injectables if necessary

Vaccinations

Vaccinations play a vital role in preventing the transmission of infectious diseases. Pharmacy technicians need to understand the stability requirements for various vaccines, which can differ based on the vaccine formulation and the manufacturer. To maintain the stability of vaccinations, pharmacy technicians should:

- Keep vaccines in a refrigerator at the suggested temperature
- Verify the expiration date before dispensing
- Dispose of any expired or improperly stored vaccines

By adhering to these guidelines for drug stability, pharmacy technicians can contribute to the safety and effectiveness of the medications they prepare and dispense.

Narrow Therapeutic Index (NTI) Medications

Narrow Therapeutic Index (NTI) medications are drugs where the gap between a beneficial dose and a harmful one is quite small. As a result, these drugs need to be administered with precision to avoid adverse effects while still achieving the desired results. Some examples of NTI medications are Warfarin, Carbamazepine, Phenytoin, Digoxin, and Lithium, which are used to treat conditions such as blood clots, seizures, heart failure, arrhythmias, and manic-depressive episodes respectively.

Pharmacy technicians play a crucial role in the safe and effective administration of these medications. They need to ensure the correct dosage is dispensed, check for potential drug interactions, monitor patients for toxicity signs or adverse effects, and report any issues to the pharmacist. It's also important for them to remind patients to follow the medication schedule as advised and report any concerns or side effects to their doctor.

Some NTI medications may require special handling or storage conditions to maintain their stability and efficacy. For instance, some may need refrigeration or protection from light. Pharmacy technicians should adhere to the manufacturer's instructions for storage and handling to maintain the medication's effectiveness. By understanding the unique challenges associated with NTI medications, pharmacy technicians can contribute to the safe and effective use of these vital drugs.

Compatibility issues during nonsterile compounding and reconstitution due to physical and chemical factors

Nonsterile compounding and reconstitution involve altering drugs to create personalized dosage forms for patients. However, this process carries a risk of physical and chemical incompatibilities between different drug ingredients, which can impact the compounded medication's stability, efficacy, and safety.

Physical incompatibilities arise when mixing two or more drugs alters the compounded medication's appearance, texture, or other physical attributes. Examples include precipitation, flocculation, or color changes.

Chemical incompatibilities occur when mixing two or more drugs triggers a chemical reaction, leading to the degradation of the drugs or the creation of new, potentially harmful compounds. Examples include hydrolysis, oxidation, or reduction.

Pharmacy technicians should be well-versed with the physical and chemical properties of the drugs they are compounding and their potential incompatibilities. They should consult reliable resources for information on drug incompatibilities and stability, verify the compatibility of ingredients before mixing, use correct techniques and equipment for accurate and uniform mixing, monitor the compounded medication for signs of physical or chemical changes and discard if necessary, and store the compounded medication as per the manufacturer's instructions with appropriate labeling.

By following these guidelines, pharmacy technicians can enhance the quality, efficacy, and safety of the compounded pharmaceuticals they produce. To ensure the safety and effectiveness of the medications they prepare, pharmacy technicians should always work under a qualified pharmacist's supervision, and some medications may require specialized training, facilities, and equipment for compounding.

Proper storage of medications

It's crucial to store medications appropriately to ensure their effectiveness, stability, and safety. Different medications have different storage needs, including specific temperature ranges, light protection, and limited access. Pharmacy technicians need to understand these storage requirements and take the necessary steps to store medications correctly.

Temperature Range

The temperature at which a medication is stored can significantly impact its stability and effectiveness. Some medications need to be kept in the fridge, while others should be stored at room temperature. If stored improperly, the chemical makeup of the medication can change, making it ineffective or even harmful.

Here are some general temperature guidelines for storing medications:

- Refrigerated medications: Keep these between 2-8°C (36-46°F) unless otherwise instructed.
- Room temperature medications: Store these between 15-30°C (59-86°F) unless otherwise instructed.
- Controlled room temperature medications: These should be kept between 20-25°C (68-77°F) unless otherwise instructed.

Light Sensitivity

Certain medications are light-sensitive and need to be protected from both direct and indirect light. Exposure to light can chemically alter the medication, reducing its effectiveness or increasing its toxicity.

Here are some general guidelines for storing light-sensitive medications:

- Protect from light medications: Store these in a dark or opaque container, away from direct or indirect light.

Restricted Access

Some medications can be harmful if misused or abused and need to be stored with limited access or special precautions to prevent unauthorized access.

Here are some general guidelines for storing restricted access medications:

- Controlled substances: These are Schedule II through Schedule V substances and legally must be stored in a locked cabinet or safe.
- Incorrectly administering high-alert drugs can have severe consequences. These should be stored separately from other medications and may need special dispensing procedures.

By adhering to these storage guidelines, pharmacy technicians can help ensure that patients receive safe and effective medications. It's important to remember that specific storage requirements can vary depending on the medication and should always be confirmed with reliable references and resources.

Chapter 6: Patient Safety and Quality of Care

High-Alert/Risk Medications and Look-Alike/Soundalike (LASA) Medications

Patients who misuse high-alert medications can face severe repercussions. It's crucial to implement strategies to prevent errors when dealing with these drugs. Medications that need continuous supervision include opioids, anticoagulants, chemotherapy drugs, insulin, and sedatives.

"Look-alike" or "sound-alike" (LASA) medications have similar names or packaging, which can easily lead to confusion among pharmacy staff. LASA errors can cause significant harm to patients. To prevent these errors, it's essential to thoroughly check labels and packaging, utilize barcode scanning technology, and set up alerts in the pharmacy management information system.

Patient safety is of utmost importance, so pharmacy technicians must be diligent in identifying LASA and high-alert drugs. By administering medication carefully and educating patients, medication errors can be prevented.

Error Prevention Strategies

In order to safeguard patient health and minimize medication errors, medical practitioners should employ a variety of techniques and strategies to prevent such mistakes. Key strategies for error prevention include:

1. Verification of Prescription or Medication Order

Before any medication is dispensed, it is crucial to confirm that a patient's details are correctly listed on the prescription or medication order. This involves checking the patient's personal information such as their name, date of birth, and address.

The verification of prescriptions or medication orders is a vital step in maintaining patient safety and avoiding medication errors. Pharmacy technicians have a significant role in this process, as they meticulously review each prescription or medication order to confirm its accuracy and suitability for the patient.

In order to validate a prescription or medication order, the technician must initially cross-check the patient's details, including their name, birth date, and address, against the information on the prescription. The prescriber's details, such as their name, contact number, and DEA number, should also be checked to ensure they are up-to-date and valid.

Next, the technician must ascertain that the ordered medication is appropriate for the patient's condition and aligns with the prescriber's instructions. This involves reviewing the details of the order, including the name of the drug, its strength, dosage form, and quantity. By evaluating the patient's medical history and current medications, the technician can identify any potential drug interactions or contraindications.

Should any inconsistencies or issues be detected during the verification process, the technician should seek further advice and clarification from the pharmacist. Once the prescription or medication order has been validated, the technician can then dispense the medication to the patient.

By diligently following these procedures and thoroughly verifying each prescription or medication order, pharmacy technicians can significantly contribute to protecting their patients from medication errors.

2. The Concept of Tall Man Lettering:

Tall Man lettering is a technique that capitalizes certain letters in medication names to help distinguish medications that look or sound alike. For instance, writing "HYDROmorphone" instead of "hydromorphone" can help avoid confusion with "morphine." This method is used to differentiate look-alike/sound-alike (LASA) medication names by capitalizing the letters that make the medication name unique. For example, to distinguish between "hydroxyzine" and "hydrALAzine," the Tall Man lettering would be "hydrOXYzine" and "hydrALAzine."

Tall Man lettering can also be used to highlight the differences between similar-looking generic and brand names. For instance, "DURagesic" (brand name) and "fentANYL" (generic name) could be written using Tall Man lettering.

This technique is an effective way to reduce medication errors caused by confusion between look-alike/sound-alike medications or similar-looking generic and brand-name medications. Pharmacy technicians should be well-versed with this error prevention strategy and ensure that medication labels and prescription orders are properly labeled with Tall Man lettering where necessary.

3. The Importance of Inventory Separation:

To prevent dispensing errors, medications with similar names or packaging should be kept separate. This includes separating look-alike and sound-alike medications.

Inventory separation is a crucial error-prevention strategy in pharmacy practice. It involves physically segregating look-alike and sound-alike (LASA) medications on the shelves, in storage, and in dispensing areas to reduce the chances of medication errors.

Inventory is separated based on medication names, dosage forms, and strengths. Similar-looking or sounding medications are stored in different sections or shelves, each labeled with the medication name and strength. For example, warfarin is separated from Coumadin, and methotrexate is separated from mitoxantrone.

Pharmacy technicians play a vital role in ensuring inventory separation by checking expiration dates, identifying similar medication names, and verifying correct storage locations. They should also report any inventory discrepancies to the pharmacist and suggest changes to improve the separation of look-alike and sound-alike medications.

By understanding the significance of inventory separation and actively monitoring it, technicians can contribute to a safer medication dispensing process.

4. Understanding Leading and Trailing Zeros:

Decimal points can be overlooked easily, so using a leading zero for values less than one and a trailing zero for whole numbers can help prevent medication dosing errors.

When dealing with numbers in medication orders or prescriptions, using leading and trailing zeros can be confusing and lead to errors. A leading zero is used before the decimal point, while a trailing zero is used after it. It's crucial to know when to use and when not to use leading and trailing zeros to avoid errors.

For numbers less than one, leading zeros are necessary, such as 0.5 mg. However, using a leading zero for a whole number, like 025 mg, is incorrect as it can be misinterpreted as 25 mg.

Trailing zeros can also cause confusion. It's incorrect to use a trailing zero when the number doesn't require one, like writing 5.0 mg instead of 5 mg. This can lead to confusion and mistakes, especially when the medication dosage is critical.

Hence, it's crucial to pay close attention to the use of leading and trailing zeros in medication orders and prescriptions to prevent errors. One way to ensure this is by using computerized physician order entry (CPOE) systems that automatically prevent leading and trailing zeros when they're not necessary.

5. Utilizing Bar Code Technology:

Bar code scanning technology is a common tool in hospitals and pharmacies to prevent the administration of incorrect medication to patients. This technology enables healthcare professionals to swiftly and precisely verify details such as the medication's name, strength, and dosage before giving it to a patient. This method is instrumental in reducing medication errors that could potentially harm patients.

Bar code technology is employed in several ways in the dispensing and administration of medication, including:

1. Medication Verification: A bar code is scanned when a patient receives their medication to ensure it is the correct one.

2. Patient Identification: All prescriptions are cross-checked with a patient's bar code before administration.

3. Inventory Management: Bar codes are used to track medication inventory and ensure that the right medications are available.

4. Order Entry: Bar codes facilitate the entry of medication orders into the electronic health record system.

The Institute for Safe Medication Practices has reported that the use of bar code technology can significantly reduce pharmaceutical errors, with hospitals seeing a 50-96% reduction in medication errors.

In addition to bar code technology, healthcare professionals should adhere to proper medication handling and administration procedures. This includes careful reading of medication labels, double-checking medication orders, and accurate documentation of medication administration.

6. Reducing the Use of Error-Prone Abbreviations:

Abbreviations can often lead to confusion or misinterpretation, making it crucial to limit their use. For instance, "q.d." (once daily) could be misinterpreted as "q.i.d." (four times daily).

Reducing the use of error-prone abbreviations is a vital strategy in preventing medication errors. While abbreviations can save time and space when writing prescriptions, they can also be misunderstood, leading to potential harm to patients.

To prevent errors caused by abbreviations, healthcare providers, including pharmaceutical technicians, should use standardized abbreviations approved by their organization. They should avoid "do not use" abbreviations that have been associated with errors, as compiled by the Joint Commission. These include abbreviations like "u" for the unit, "IU" for the international unit, and "MS" for morphine sulfate.

In addition to using standardized abbreviations, healthcare providers should communicate clearly when writing prescriptions or medication orders. They should avoid using abbreviations or medical jargon that may be unfamiliar to the patient or other healthcare team members. Clear and simple language, along with detailed instructions, should be used to ensure the patient receives the correct medication in the appropriate dosage and frequency.

By implementing these methods, pharmacy technicians and other medical staff can contribute significantly to ensuring patient safety and preventing drug errors.

Issues that require pharmacist intervention

The role of a pharmacist is crucial in patient care and improving the results of pharmaceutical treatments. They are often called upon to address issues such as drug utilization review (DUR), adverse drug events (ADEs), over-the-counter (OTC) suggestions, therapeutic substitutions, misuse of medication, patient adherence to medication, post-vaccination follow-ups, drug interactions, and allergies.

DUR is a method used by pharmacists to analyze a patient's medication regimen to identify potential problems like drug interactions, repeated therapy, and incorrect dosage. Pharmacists use resources like electronic health records and medication databases to carry out DUR and provide appropriate advice to prescribers.

ADEs are any harmful or unintended consequences of a drug. Pharmacists can prevent and manage ADEs by monitoring patients for potential side effects, educating them on medication usage, and suggesting alternative treatments.

Pharmacists can also provide OTC suggestions for patients who are looking for self-care options for minor health issues. This could involve recommending a suitable OTC product, advising on correct usage and dosage, and monitoring for potential side effects.

Therapeutic substitutions are when an alternative medication is used to achieve the same therapeutic effect as the initially prescribed drug. Pharmacists may suggest therapeutic substitutions when a cheaper or more effective medication is available, or when a patient has an adverse reaction to the original medication.

Medication misuse can happen due to incorrect dosage, delivery, or storage. Pharmacists can help reduce drug abuse by educating patients about safe medication handling and storage and recognizing early signs of misuse.

Adherence refers to a patient's ability to follow their medication regimen as prescribed. Poor adherence can result in treatment failure and negative outcomes. Pharmacists can improve adherence by providing education on medication use, identifying and addressing barriers to adherence, and offering tools like pill organizers or reminders.

Post-vaccination follow-up involves monitoring patients for potential side effects after immunization. Pharmacists play a crucial role in this by educating patients on common side effects and monitoring for potential adverse events.

Allergies and drug interactions are serious issues that may require a pharmacist's intervention. Pharmacists can help identify potential allergies or drug interactions through medication reconciliation and reviewing the patient's medical history. They can also suggest alternative treatments or dosage adjustments to prevent negative outcomes.

Pharmacists play a vital role in identifying and addressing medication-related issues to ensure patient safety and improve medication therapy outcomes.

Drug Utilization Review [DUR]

Pharmacists play a crucial role in ensuring patient safety and improving medication therapy outcomes. One key tool they use to identify potential drug-related issues is DUR. DUR involves reviewing patient medication profiles to identify potential issues related to medication therapy, such as drug interactions, duplications, allergies, and inappropriate dosages.

Pharmacy technicians support pharmacists during the DUR process. Their tasks may include updating patient medication profiles, conducting medication histories, and reviewing prescription orders for accuracy and completeness.

Understanding the concept of DUR and its application in pharmacy practice is important for pharmacy technicians. On the PTCB exam, you may be asked about DUR and its role in ensuring patient safety. You may also be asked to identify potential drug-related problems and suggest suitable interventions for pharmacists to consider.

Adverse Drug Event [ADE]

ADEs are unintended and harmful outcomes that can occur from medication use. These events can range from mild side effects to life-threatening reactions. Some ADEs can be prevented or reduced with appropriate pharmacist intervention. Pharmacy technicians play a crucial role in identifying ADEs and alerting the pharmacist to take suitable action.

Common ADEs include allergic reactions, gastrointestinal issues, respiratory problems, cardiovascular problems, and central nervous system problems.

Pharmacists can take several steps to avoid or reduce the severity of ADEs. They can review the patient's past medications to identify any interactions or other risks. They can adjust medication doses or switch to alternative medications to reduce the risk of ADEs. They can also educate patients on safe medication use and monitor for signs of ADEs.

As a pharmacy technician, it's your responsibility to recognize the symptoms of ADEs and immediately inform your pharmacist if you suspect a patient is experiencing one. This can help prevent severe harm and ensure that patients receive appropriate care.

Over-The-Counter (OTC) Medication Advice

Many people use over-the-counter (OTC) drugs to manage common health issues like allergies, pain, colds, and flu. Pharmacists play a vital role in guiding patients on the correct use of these products to guarantee their safety and effectiveness. There are several areas where a pharmacist's intervention may be necessary when recommending OTC medications:

1. Drug Interactions: OTC drugs can sometimes interact with prescription medications, resulting in severe health problems. For instance, taking aspirin alongside blood-thinning drugs can increase the risk of bleeding. Pharmacists should be aware of potential drug interactions to provide appropriate advice to patients.

2. Side Effects: OTC drugs can cause side effects such as stomach upset, allergic reactions, and drowsiness. Pharmacists should guide patients

on how to recognize and manage these side effects and when to seek medical help.

3. Age Restrictions: Certain OTC drugs are not suitable for specific age groups. For instance, aspirin should not be administered to children under 12 due to the risk of Reye's syndrome. Pharmacists should be knowledgeable about these age restrictions and advise patients accordingly.

4. Pregnancy and Breastfeeding: Some OTC drugs may be harmful during pregnancy and breastfeeding. Pharmacists should guide patients on the safe use of OTC drugs during these periods and suggest alternative treatments when necessary.

5. Misuse: OTC drugs can be misused, leading to serious health issues. For example, frequent use of nasal decongestants can result in rebound congestion. Pharmacists should educate patients on the safe use of OTC drugs and discourage misuse.

In summary, pharmacists have a crucial role in ensuring patients reap the benefits of OTC drugs while minimizing potential risks. They need to intervene in cases of drug interactions, side effects, age restrictions, pregnancy and breastfeeding, and misuse.

Therapeutic Substitution

Therapeutic substitution involves replacing one drug with another that is expected to have similar therapeutic effects. This can happen for various reasons like cost-saving, drug shortages, or changes in medication formulary. Before making a therapeutic substitution, the pharmacist must review the patient's medical history, current medication regimen, and potential drug interactions.

For instance, a patient may be using a brand-name drug for a specific condition, but the pharmacy only has the generic version. The pharmacist may need to make a therapeutic substitution to provide the patient with a similar drug. However, the pharmacist must consider any potential differences in bioavailability, potency, and side effects between the brand-name and generic drug.

Pharmacy technicians should understand the process of therapeutic substitution and be able to communicate any changes to the patient or healthcare provider. They also need to be aware of the risks of therapeutic substitution and the importance of double-checking prescriptions before dispensing.

Misuse

Misuse refers to the incorrect use of medication, not following the doctor's instructions or the directions on the drug label. Misuse can include taking too much, taking it at the wrong time, or using an unprescribed drug. Misuse can lead to harmful drug reactions or other negative health outcomes, so pharmacists have a crucial role in identifying and managing overuse.

Pharmacists can help prevent medication misuse by advising patients on the correct use of their drugs, including dosage instructions, timing, and potential side effects. They may also need to collaborate with prescribers to adjust medication regimens or suggest alternative drugs to better meet the patients' needs and reduce the risk of misuse.

Adherence

Adherence is a crucial issue that requires pharmacist intervention to ensure patients take their medications as prescribed. Poor adherence can result in several negative outcomes, including treatment failure, disease progression, and increased healthcare costs. Pharmacists play a vital role in identifying and addressing adherence issues through various strategies, including patient education, medication therapy management, and using adherence aids like pillboxes and reminder apps.

Pharmacists can work with patients to identify the specific barriers to adherence and develop strategies to overcome them. This may involve simplifying the dosing schedule, switching to a different medication with fewer side effects, or connecting patients with financial assistance programs.

Pharmacists can also use various tools and techniques to monitor and improve adherence. For example, they may conduct medication reviews to ensure that patients take their medications correctly and identify potential drug interactions. They may also use electronic health records to track patients' medication adherence over time and identify patients needing additional support or interventions.

Overall, ensuring medication adherence is critical to patient safety and quality assurance, and pharmacists play a crucial role in promoting adherence and preventing medication-related problems.

Post-Immunization Follow-Up

Pharmacists play a key role in patient safety, especially in monitoring for possible side effects after a patient has been immunized. These side effects can vary from mild symptoms like pain, swelling, fever, and general discomfort to severe reactions such as allergies or anaphylaxis.

It's important for pharmacists to be well-versed in the recommended immunization schedule and the correct methods of administering vaccines. This ensures that patients receive the right vaccine at the right time. Pharmacists also need to understand the potential side effects of each vaccine and what to do if a patient has an adverse reaction.

Follow-up care after immunization is a crucial part of patient care, and pharmacists play a significant role in this. They may be responsible for monitoring patients for any adverse reactions, providing appropriate advice and care if a patient experiences a side effect or an adverse reaction after immunization.

In situations where a patient has a severe adverse reaction, pharmacists may need to collaborate with other healthcare providers to ensure the patient gets the right care and treatment. By providing comprehensive follow-up care after immunization, pharmacists can help ensure that patients fully benefit from immunization while minimizing the risk of adverse effects.

Allergies

Allergies are a common problem that often requires the intervention of a pharmacist. A patient with a known allergy to a certain medication can have an adverse reaction, which can be life-threatening in severe cases. Pharmacists need to be aware of a patient's allergies to ensure that the prescribed medication does not contain any allergens. If a medication that contains a potential allergen is prescribed, the pharmacist must inform the prescriber and collaborate with them to find a safe alternative medication for the patient. In some situations, the pharmacist may also need to educate the patient about the potential risks of taking a medication that contains an allergen and provide advice on managing any adverse reactions. Additionally, the pharmacist may need to update the patient's medication history and allergy information in their records to prevent future incidents.

Drug Interactions

Drug interactions occur when two or more medications interact in the body, leading to unexpected side effects or a decrease in the effectiveness of one or both drugs. This can happen when different medications are taken together or even when certain foods or supplements are consumed while taking medication.

Pharmacists play a crucial role in identifying potential drug interactions and preventing harmful effects. They can examine a patient’s medication regimen and health history to determine if any potential drug interactions may occur. In some cases, the pharmacist may suggest adjusting the medication dosage or switching to a different medication to avoid harmful interactions.

Patients should always inform their healthcare provider about their medications, supplements, and vitamins to help identify potential drug interactions. Pharmacy technicians must be aware of this issue and assist patients in providing this information to their healthcare providers.

Additionally, pharmacists can use computer software programs to screen for potential drug interactions, alerting them to any issues that may arise. This technology, combined with a pharmacist’s clinical knowledge and experience, can help ensure patient safety and prevent adverse drug interactions.

Event reporting procedures

The procedures for reporting events are vital for maintaining patient safety and avoiding medication errors. Such procedures encompass reporting medication mistakes, adverse reactions, and issues with product integrity to the relevant authorities. MedWatch, a voluntary reporting system overseen by the Food and Drug Administration (FDA), is a crucial tool for reporting adverse events.

Near-miss incidents also form a significant part of incident reporting. These are situations where the patient could have been harmed but wasn't. It's essential to report these near misses to prevent similar incidents from happening in the future.

A method known as root-cause analysis (RCA) can help prevent medication errors and other adverse outcomes. This involves examining the entire patient care process, from diagnosis to administration, to identify potential causes of the error. Once the causes are identified, steps can be taken to prevent the same issue from recurring.

Pharmacy technicians play a vital role in event reporting procedures. They are often the first to spot potential medication errors or adverse events and should report these incidents to their supervisors or other relevant authorities immediately. It's crucial for pharmacy technicians to understand the importance of event reporting and be familiar with the incident reporting procedures.

Medication Errors

Medication errors, due to the serious risk they pose to patients, must be reported so they can be addressed and eliminated. Medication errors can involve anything that could result in a patient receiving the wrong medication or experiencing any other type of harm. Errors can occur at any stage in the medication-use process, from prescribing to dispensing to administration to monitoring.

Pharmacists play a key role in identifying and reporting medication errors, but as a pharmacy technician, you may also be involved in this process. It's essential to report medication errors to prevent similar mistakes from happening in the future. As a pharmacy technician, you should report medication errors to your supervisor or the pharmacist in charge without delay.

When reporting a medication error, you should include the following details:

- The patient's name and identification information
- The name and strength of the medication
- The form and route of administration of the dosage
- The date and time the error happened
- The nature of the error and the harm caused
- Any factors or circumstances contributing to the error
- Any corrective actions taken to prevent the error from happening again

Reporting medication errors is a crucial aspect of quality assurance and patient safety. It allows healthcare professionals to identify error patterns, take corrective action to prevent future errors, and ultimately enhance patient outcomes.

Adverse Effects

Adverse effects are any unintended and harmful effects of medication or treatment experienced by a patient. These effects can range from mild to severe and can affect any part of the body. Adverse effects can happen for various reasons, such as medication interactions, allergic reactions, dosage errors, or other medical conditions. It's crucial to promptly report any adverse effects to a pharmacist.

Pharmacists play a key role in identifying, reporting, and managing adverse effects. They may sometimes need to alter the patient's medication dosage or switch to a different medication to reduce adverse effects. It's important to note that adverse effects may not be immediately noticeable after starting a medication. They can happen at any time during treatment, so it's important to monitor changes in a patient's health condition and report any concerns promptly.

Reporting adverse effects is a crucial part of patient safety and quality assurance. Pharmacists and pharmacy technicians should be familiar with the reporting procedures and guidelines set by regulatory bodies like the FDA and MedWatch. Adverse effects should be reported promptly, and necessary measures should be taken to ensure the patient's safety and well-being. Failure to report adverse effects can lead to serious consequences and put the patient's health at risk.

Product Integrity

The process of reporting events is crucial in ensuring the safety of patients and maintaining the quality of pharmaceutical products. The term "product integrity" pertains to the state and authenticity of pharmaceutical items, which can be jeopardized during production, storage, and distribution. Any suspected or verified issues with product integrity must be reported to the relevant regulatory body or manufacturer to facilitate immediate investigation and suitable corrective measures.

Pharmacy technicians should also report any adverse effects that patients experience while using these products. An adverse effect is any unintended and harmful reaction to a medication or pharmaceutical product. These effects can range from minor to severe and can be caused by various factors, such as drug interactions, allergic reactions, or errors in medication. Reporting these adverse effects can aid in identifying product safety issues and preventing harm to patients.

Errors in prescribing, dispensing, or administering a medication should also be reported by pharmacy technicians. This reporting can help enhance the process of drug usage and decrease the chances of future medication errors that could potentially harm patients.

The U.S. Food and Drug Administration (FDA) operates a program called MedWatch, which allows healthcare providers and patients to report adverse events associated with pharmaceutical products. Pharmacy technicians can use this system to report incidents. Other reporting systems may include internal mechanisms within the pharmacy, such as a near-miss reporting system that reports and investigates events that could potentially harm patients but have not yet done so. Root cause analysis (RCA) is another reporting procedure that identifies the fundamental causes of an event to prevent it from happening again.

Understanding these reporting procedures and reporting any events promptly and accurately is vital for pharmacy technicians to ensure patient safety and the quality of pharmaceutical products.

MedWatch

The FDA's MedWatch program encourages the reporting of medication errors, quality issues, and side effects of prescription and over-the-counter drugs, biologics, medical devices, nutritional supplements, and cosmetics. The FDA runs this essential program to ensure the quality and safety of healthcare products available to consumers.

Pharmacy technicians play a crucial role in recognizing and reporting adverse events or product quality issues to MedWatch. They should advise patients to report any side effects or quality issues with their medications, and they should report any unusual occurrences during the dispensing, administering, or storage of pharmaceuticals. Pharmacy technicians should be familiar with the reporting requirements, including the information needed for a report, and the process of submitting it to the FDA.

In conclusion, MedWatch plays a vital role in monitoring the effectiveness and safety of medical supplies and pharmaceuticals. Pharmacy technicians should be familiar with the program and encourage patients to report any adverse events or product quality issues. They should also be aware of the reporting requirements and the process of submitting reports to the FDA.

Near Miss Reporting

The establishment of event reporting protocols is crucial for ensuring patient safety and maintaining quality standards in a pharmacy environment. One such event that necessitates reporting is a near miss. This term refers to an incident that could have potentially harmed the patient, but did not.

In the event of a near miss, it is the responsibility of pharmacy technicians to promptly inform their superiors or the designated reporting system. The reporting of near misses facilitates the recognition of potential risks and the development of strategies to avert similar occurrences in the future.

When documenting a near miss, pharmacy technicians should include as many details as possible. This should encompass information such as the date and time of the incident, the people involved, and a comprehensive description of the event. Identifying the root cause of the near miss is also crucial as it aids in pinpointing areas that need improvement in the pharmacy's operations and procedures.

The reporting of near misses is a critical aspect of patient safety and quality assurance in a pharmacy setting. Pharmacy technicians must understand the importance of reporting near misses and always prioritize patient safety.

Root-Cause Analysis (RCA)

Medication errors and adverse drug reactions are two instances where a root-cause analysis (RCA) can be conducted to ascertain what went wrong and how to prevent it from happening again. RCA is a vital tool for improving healthcare quality and reducing patient risks.

The RCA process usually entails several steps, such as:

1. Event Identification: This involves documenting the incident and collecting all pertinent data, including patient details, medication specifics, and other relevant information.

2. Team Formation: A team of individuals with expertise in the area of the incident is formed to carry out the RCA. This team generally consists of pharmacy technicians, pharmacists, doctors, and other healthcare professionals.

3. Event Investigation: The team scrutinizes all the available information and conducts interviews with the staff involved in the incident. This assists in identifying the root causes of the event.

4. Root Cause Identification: Based on the investigation, the team pinpoints the root causes of the incident. These could be due to communication failures, system breakdowns, or human error.

5. Corrective Action Plan Development: The team formulates a plan to address the root causes of the incident and prevent similar incidents in the future. This could involve modifications to policies and procedures, further training, or other measures.

6. Corrective Action Implementation: The team executes the corrective actions and monitors the effectiveness of these interventions.

By employing RCA to identify and address the root causes of medication errors and adverse drug reactions, pharmacy technicians and other healthcare professionals can enhance patient safety and prevent future mistakes.

Types of prescription errors

Categories of Prescription Mistakes:

Incorrect Dosages:

These types of errors happen when a patient is given a dosage that is either too high or too low, which can lead to potential harm or ineffective treatment. This could be a result of misreading or misunderstanding the prescription, or a miscalculation in the preparation of the medication.

Incorrect dosages are prescription mistakes that involve the wrong amount of medication. This can encompass giving a patient an excessive or insufficient amount of medication and incorrect intervals between dosages. Various factors, such as confusion between metric and non-metric units, misinterpretation of handwritten prescriptions, or miscalculation of dosages, can lead to incorrect dosages.

Pharmacy technicians need to be aware of the potential for incorrect dosages and implement measures to avoid them. This could include double-checking calculations, confirming the prescribed dose with the prescriber if it seems unusual, and ensuring that it is suitable for the patient's age, weight, and medical condition.

Pharmacy technicians should also understand the potential risks associated with incorrect dosages. Overdoses can result in adverse drug reactions, while underdoses may lead to ineffective treatment. In some cases, incorrect dosages can even be life-threatening, emphasizing the crucial importance of accurate dosing.

Premature Refills:

This type of error happens when a patient gets a medication refill before the due time, which could lead to misuse, abuse, or potential harm. This could be due to a miscommunication between the prescriber and the pharmacy or a misunderstanding by the patient.

Premature refill errors happen when a prescription is filled before the due date, leading to potential overdoses or drug interactions. These errors can be caused by several factors, including misunderstanding of the prescription, errors in calculation, or pressure to fulfill the prescription as soon as possible.

Pharmacy technicians play a vital role in identifying and preventing premature refill errors. One way they can do this is by checking prescription records to ensure that a prescription is being filled at the right time. Another method is communicating with the pharmacist and the patient to clarify any confusion or concerns about the prescription.

Any premature refill errors should be reported immediately to the prescribing doctor or pharmacist. If the patient is taking the medication, they should stop until the issue is resolved. Implementing more safety checks in the filling process and improving communication with prescribers are two additional steps that can be taken to reduce the likelihood of future errors.

Mistake in Medication Quantity:

This error happens when a patient is given an incorrect amount of medication, which could potentially harm them or render the treatment ineffective. This could be a result of an error in calculating or preparing the medication, or a misunderstanding of the prescription.

This type of error is common when a pharmacy technician is filling a prescription. It could occur in several ways, such as miscounting pills or incorrectly measuring liquid medications.

If a patient is given the wrong amount of medication, the consequences could be severe. The medication might not work as intended, or the patient could suffer from side effects due to an overdose or underdose. This is particularly worrying for patients with chronic conditions who need consistent dosing for the best health results.

To avoid such errors, pharmacy technicians should be extra careful when counting or measuring medications. They should also verify their work before giving the medication to the pharmacist for final approval. If there's any confusion or uncertainty about the prescribed quantity, they should always seek clarification from the pharmacist or the person who prescribed the medication.

By adhering to these best practices, pharmacy technicians can ensure that patients always receive the correct amount of medication.

Mistake in Patient Identity:

This error happens when a patient is given medication meant for another patient, which could potentially harm them or render the treatment ineffective. This could be a result of misreading or misunderstanding the prescription, or a mix-up in the pharmacy's computer system or physical inventory.

Giving medication to the wrong patient is a potentially dangerous mistake with serious consequences. This type of error could occur when the prescriber enters incorrect patient information into the electronic health record, or when a pharmacy technician selects the wrong medication for a patient with a similar name. It's crucial to avoid this error by double-checking patient identification before dispensing medications and confirming patient information with the prescriber if there's any confusion. Additionally, pharmacy technicians should always ensure that the medication label matches the prescription and includes the correct patient name and identifying information. If a prescription error is detected, it should be reported immediately to prevent harm to the patient.

Mistake in Medication Type:

This error happens when a patient is given a different medication than the one prescribed, which could potentially harm them or render the treatment ineffective. This could be a result of misreading or misunderstanding the prescription, or a mix-up in the pharmacy's computer system or physical inventory.

An error in medication type occurs when the wrong medication is dispensed to the patient. Various factors can cause this type of error, such as medications that look or sound alike, misinterpretation of the prescription, or incorrect entry of the medication into the computer system. Errors in medication type can have serious consequences, such as adverse drug reactions, drug interactions, or even death.

To avoid such errors, pharmacy technicians must verify the prescription with the prescriber, double-check the medication label and packaging, and confirm the drug with the patient. Additionally, being aware of medications that look or sound alike and understanding drug indications, dosages, and administration routes is crucial. Any discrepancies or concerns should be immediately reported to the pharmacist or prescriber to prevent harm to the patient.

Hygiene and cleaning standards

Pharmacy technicians have the responsibility of ensuring a hazard-free workplace. The importance of hygiene and cleanliness cannot be overstated, as they are key in preventing the spread of harmful microbes. Regular cleaning of counting trays, counters, and equipment is necessary, and personal protective equipment (PPE) such as gloves and masks should be utilized when required.

Handwashing is a simple but highly effective measure to prevent disease transmission. It is essential to wash hands thoroughly with soap and water for a minimum of 20/25 seconds before and after handling any medication, and after using the restroom or blowing your nose. If soap and water are not available, hand sanitizer with at least 60% alcohol can be used as an alternative.

PPE like gloves and masks can also help prevent germ transmission. Gloves should be changed frequently and disposed of correctly, while masks should be worn when there's a risk of respiratory droplets.

Besides personal hygiene, maintaining a clean and uncontaminated pharmacy environment is crucial. Regular cleaning of counting trays, countertops, and equipment with disinfectant solutions is necessary. It's also important to adhere to any specific cleaning protocols set by the pharmacy or manufacturer. By adhering to these hygiene and cleaning standards, pharmacy technicians can help ensure their safety and that of their patients.

Handwashing

Hygiene and cleaning standards are vital for ensuring a safe and clean pharmacy environment. Handwashing is a significant and effective method to prevent infection spread. Pharmacy technicians should wash their hands thoroughly with soap and water for at least 20 seconds before and after handling medication, equipment, or patient interaction.

Apart from handwashing, pharmacy technicians should also adhere to other hygiene and cleaning standards to prevent germ spread. This could include wearing PPE like masks and gloves when necessary. Technicians should also regularly clean and disinfect counting trays, countertops, and equipment and properly dispose of any contaminated materials or waste.

For the safety and cleanliness of their environment, it's imperative for pharmacy technicians to understand and follow hygiene and cleaning standards for themselves, their colleagues, and their patients.

Personal protective equipment (PPE)

PPE is crucial for maintaining hygiene and cleanliness in the pharmacy. PPE includes items like gloves, gowns, masks, and eyewear, which are designed to protect the wearer from potential hazards such as exposure to infectious agents or harmful chemicals.

When handling medications or other products in the pharmacy, wearing the appropriate PPE is essential. Gloves should be worn when handling medications or touching potentially contaminated surfaces. Gowns or lab coats should be worn to protect clothing from contamination. Masks and eyewear may be necessary when working with hazardous chemicals or procedures that generate airborne particles.

Proper donning and doffing of PPE to prevent contamination is essential. Hands should be thoroughly washed before and after putting on or removing PPE, and care should be taken to avoid touching any contaminated surfaces. PPE should be properly disposed of after use and should never be reused.

Adherence to proper hygiene and cleaning standards, including the use of PPE, is crucial for maintaining a safe and clean pharmacy environment and protecting patients and staff from potential harm.

Keeping Counting Trays Clean

In a pharmacy, it's crucial to uphold strict cleanliness and hygiene standards to safeguard patient health. One key aspect of this involves the regular cleaning of medication counting trays. After each use, these trays should be washed using soap and water, thoroughly rinsed, and then sanitized with a suitable solution such as 70% isopropyl alcohol or bleach. The tray must be fully air-dried before it's used again. To avoid cross-contamination, it's equally important to clean the immediate workspace, including the countertop and any equipment used. Regular handwashing and the use of hand sanitizer when soap and water aren't readily available are also fundamental in maintaining a clean and safe workspace. Pharmacy staff should also wear protective gear like gloves and masks to prevent infection spread.

Keeping Countertops Clean

Pharmacy countertops play a significant role in safeguarding patient health and preventing disease transmission. Regular cleaning and disinfection of these surfaces are vital in maintaining a clean and sterile workspace. Here are some steps to clean the countertop:

1. Start by clearing all items from the countertop, including equipment, supplies, and medication.

2. Discard any used materials, like cotton swabs or medication vials.

3. Clean the countertop using a mild detergent and warm water, wiping away any spills or debris.

4. Rinse the countertop thoroughly with clean water to remove all detergent residue.

5. Use a hospital-grade disinfectant spray or wipe to disinfect the countertop, following the manufacturer's instructions for application and contact time.

6. Allow the countertop to fully air dry before replacing any items.

Regular countertop cleaning, especially after each use, is crucial to prevent cross-contamination and maintain a clean and safe workspace for pharmacy technicians and their patients.

Equipment Hygiene

Maintaining cleanliness and hygiene in a pharmacy is crucial to prevent infection spread and ensure patient safety. Proper cleaning of equipment used in medication preparation, like pill counters and mixing devices, is vital to avoid cross-contamination and potential incorrect dosage contamination. Following the manufacturer's guidelines for cleaning and maintaining equipment, including using suitable cleaning solutions and disinfectants, is essential.

When handling drugs or preparing prescriptions, it's also important to use personal protective equipment (PPE). This includes gloves, masks, and gowns. Gloves should be worn at all times when administering medication and changed between patients to prevent disease transmission. Masks should be worn in areas where airborne pathogens may be present or when preparing sterile pharmaceuticals. Gowns and eye protection should be worn when there's a risk of exposure to bodily fluids or other hazardous materials.

Countertops should be regularly cleaned and disinfected to prevent bacteria and other microorganisms' growth. A solution of water and a disinfectant cleaner should be used to wipe down countertops, and any spills or stains should be promptly cleaned. It's crucial to avoid using harsh chemicals that may damage the countertop surface or leave a residue that could contaminate medications.

Upholding hygiene and cleanliness standards is crucial to ensuring patient safety in a pharmacy setting. By adhering to proper cleaning procedures for equipment, using PPE, and disinfecting surfaces, pharmacy technicians can help prevent infection spread and foster a safe and healthy environment for patients and staff.

Chapter 7: Order Entry and Processing

Methods for preparing non-sterile formulations

The role of a pharmacy technician involves the crucial task of preparing non-sterile pharmaceutical products. These items can range from ointments and mixtures to liquids, emulsions, suppositories, and enemas. Such products are often prescribed by healthcare professionals to cater to the unique needs of each patient.

When creating these non-sterile products, it's imperative for pharmacy technicians to adhere to specific procedures to guarantee accuracy, safety, and effectiveness. These procedures can involve choosing the correct ingredients and tools, accurately measuring and combining ingredients, and ensuring the final product aligns with established quality guidelines.

Certain non-sterile products may require specialized techniques during their preparation. For instance, when creating ointments, a mortar and pestle might be needed to achieve the desired consistency. In the case of suppositories, molds are used to form the correct shape and size.

Being well-versed in the processes used to prepare non-sterile products and the best practices for ensuring their quality and safety is a must for pharmacy technicians. By adhering to established procedures and guidelines, they can help guarantee that patients receive the best care possible.

Ointments

Ointments are semi-solid substances that are applied directly to the skin. They can be medicinal or non-medicinal and are typically composed of oils, waxes, and water. Ointments are commonly used to treat various skin conditions, such as eczema, psoriasis, and minor injuries.

The process of compounding ointments requires precise measurements and meticulous attention to detail. The general procedures followed include:

1. Accurately weighing and measuring all ingredients using a calibrated scale and measuring tools.

2. Melting solid ingredients like wax in a double boiler or microwave until they are fully melted and transparent.

3. Gradually adding liquid ingredients like oil to the melted wax while continuously stirring to form a uniform mixture.

4. Thoroughly mixing in any active pharmaceutical ingredients or additional additives as per the prescription or formula.

5. Transferring the mixture into a suitable container, such as a jar or tube, and allowing it to cool to room temperature.

6. Labeling the container with the patient's name, the name and strength of the medication, and the date of compounding.

Maintaining cleanliness and good hygiene during the compounding process is crucial to prevent contamination and ensure patient safety. This involves using appropriate personal protective equipment (PPE), such as gloves and a lab coat, and thoroughly cleaning all surfaces and tools before and after compounding.

Mixtures

When preparing non-sterile products like mixtures, following the correct procedures is vital to ensure accuracy, safety, and quality. The steps typically involved in compounding mixtures include:

1. Calculating the quantity of each ingredient based on the prescribed dosage and strength.

2. Checking for potential drug interactions and allergies, and verifying that the medication is suitable for the patient.

3. Accurately weighing or measuring each ingredient, and recording the quantities used.

4. Combining the ingredients in the correct sequence and mixing thoroughly to ensure uniformity.

5. Labeling the final product with the necessary information, including the patient's name, the name and strength of the medication, dosage, and expiration date.

Besides these general steps, specific procedures may be required for certain mixtures, such as suspensions or solutions. It's crucial for pharmacy technicians to be familiar with these procedures and to follow them diligently to ensure patient safety and accurate medication dispensing.

Making Non-Sterile Liquids

When creating non-sterile liquids like compounded medications, it's vital to be precise and careful to ensure the end product is safe and effective. Here are the steps to follow:

1. Determine the required amounts: Start by figuring out the exact quantities of each ingredient needed for the mixture. This ensures that the final product has the right proportions of each component.

2. Choose the right tools: Select equipment that's suitable for the volume and thickness of the liquid you're compounding. This could include graduated cylinders, beakers, or mixing containers.

3. Get the ingredients ready: Measure each ingredient accurately and transfer them into the mixing container.

4. Combine the ingredients: Stir the ingredients until they're evenly mixed. You might need to use a stir bar or magnetic stirrer for this.

5. Test the pH: Depending on the recipe, you might need to adjust the pH of the solution to ensure it's stable and suitable for the patient.

6. Package the final product: Once the product is compounded and quality-checked, it should be appropriately labeled and packaged.

It's crucial to adhere to standard procedures and keep your workspace clean and organized when making non-sterile products to ensure patient safety and regulatory compliance.

Creating Non-Sterile Emulsions

When making non-sterile products like emulsions, it's essential to follow specific protocols to ensure the final product is safe and effective. Here are the steps:

1. Clean and sanitize all tools and surfaces that will touch the ingredients and final product.

2. Accurately weigh and measure all ingredients, following the prescriber's formula and instructions.

3. Mix the oil-based and water-based ingredients separately, heating and stirring as needed to ensure they're fully combined and dissolved.

4. Gradually add the oil mixture to the water mixture, stirring constantly to create an emulsion.

5. Continue stirring until the oil and water phases no longer separate and the emulsion is fully formed.

6. Transfer the final product to a clean, sterile container and label it with the name, strength, and expiration date.

It's also important to regularly check and record the product's temperature and pH during the compounding process to ensure they stay within acceptable ranges. Any deviations or discrepancies should be immediately addressed and documented.

Making Non-Sterile Suppositories

Suppositories are small, solid, bullet-shaped doses designed for rectal or vaginal insertion. They deliver medication directly to the required area, bypassing the digestive system and liver. Suppositories can be compounded in various shapes and sizes, depending on the patient's needs.

To make a non-sterile suppository, start by choosing the right base. Suppository bases can include cocoa butter, hydrogenated vegetable oil, and glycerinated gelatin. Melt the base over low heat in a double boiler until it reaches a temperature of about 45-50°C.

Next, add the active ingredient or ingredients to the melted base. These could include pain relievers, anti-nausea drugs, or hormones. Mix the active ingredient thoroughly into the base to ensure even distribution.

Once the active ingredient is mixed in, pour the mixture into a suppository mold. Prep the mold by lightly coating the inside with a lubricant like mineral oil to make it easier to remove the finished suppositories. Fill the mold to the desired level and scrape off any excess mixture from the top with a spatula.

Put the filled mold in a refrigerator or freezer to let the suppositories harden. Once they're solid, they can be removed from the mold and stored in a cool, dry place until needed. Don't forget to label the suppositories with the medication's name, strength, and expiration date.

Enemas Preparation

The process of preparing enemas is a routine job for pharmacy technicians. Enemas are used for multiple reasons, including bowel cleansing, administering medication, and carrying out diagnostic tests. Here are the general steps to prepare a non-sterile enema:

1. Collect all the required materials and equipment: You'll need an enema bag or bottle, a catheter or nozzle, warm water, the medication prescribed by the doctor, and any other necessary items like lubricant, gloves, or syringes.

2. Work out the correct dosage of medication: To figure out the right amount of medication for a patient, you'll need to use a formula that takes into account the dosage recommended by the doctor and the patient's weight.

3. Combine the medication with warm water in a sterile container until it's completely dissolved. If the medication needs to be diluted, measure the right amount of sterile water for this.

4. Add the prepared medication to the enema bag or bottle: Once the medication is ready, put it in the enema bag or bottle. Make sure to get rid of any air bubbles in the bag or bottle to avoid causing discomfort during the procedure.

5. Get the patient ready: Make sure the patient is comfortable, typically lying on their left side with their knees bent.

6. Give the enema: Apply lubricant to the catheter or nozzle and gently insert it into the rectum, being careful not to cause any discomfort. Slowly squeeze the bag or bottle to deliver the medication into the patient's rectum. It's important to keep an eye on the patient's comfort level while doing this.

7. Dispose of the materials: After the enema has been given, all materials should be disposed of properly in line with local regulations.

The process of preparing enemas may vary slightly depending on the medication and the patient's condition. Pharmacy technicians should always adhere to their facility's rules and procedures for preparing non-sterile products to ensure the safety of the patient and the correct administration of the medication.

Formulas, proportions, alligations, calculations, ratios, conversions, Sig codes

Pharmacy technicians involved in the compounding of medications need to have a comprehensive understanding of various formulas and calculations to ensure the accurate preparation of medication

doses and concentrations. Here are some standard formulas used in pharmacy compounding:

- Alligation: This formula is used to determine the quantity of two or more solutions of varying strengths that need to be mixed to achieve a specific strength. This is a common practice in medication compounding.
- Ratio and Proportion: This formula is used to identify the relationship between two or more quantities. It is often used to figure out the quantity of medication to be dispensed based on the patient's weight.
- Dilution: This formula is used to calculate the precise amount of a stock solution required to prepare a desired concentration of a diluted solution. This is frequently used in medication compounding.

Pharmacy technicians need to understand various calculations, ratios, and proportions used in pharmacy practice. Here are some of the most common calculations and formulas:

- Dosage calculations: To calculate the correct medication dosage, technicians need information on the patient's weight, the strength of the medication, and the desired dosage. The formula for calculating dosage is: Dosage = (Weight x Desired Dose) / Strength of Medication.
- Dilution calculations: These calculations are used to determine the quantity of medication required to achieve a specific concentration. The formula for dilution is (Amount of Stock Solution) / (Amount of Diluted Solution) = (Concentration of Diluted Solution) / (Concentration of Stock Solution).

- Alligations: These are used to calculate the ratio of two solutions of varying strengths mixed to create a solution of a specific strength. Pharmacy technicians use alligations to figure out the correct ratio of two solutions to mix. There are two types of alligations: weighted and unweighted.

In addition to these formulas, pharmacy technicians need to be familiar with various medical abbreviations and symbols commonly used in prescriptions, such as:

- Sig Codes: These are instructions for medication intake, often including Latin abbreviations. For instance, B.I.D. (twice daily), T.I.D. (three times daily), Q.I.D. (four times daily), A.C. (before meals), and P.C. (after meals).
- Medical Terminology: This refers to the language used to describe medical conditions, procedures, and medications. Pharmacy technicians need to understand medical terminology to accurately interpret prescriptions and communicate with other healthcare professionals. Examples include PO (by mouth), IM (intramuscular), IV (intravenous), QD (once daily), PRN (as needed), and Disp (dispense).
- Days Supply: This refers to the duration for which a medication will last. Pharmacy technicians need to be able to calculate the day's supply to label the medication accurately.
- Quantity: Pharmacy technicians need to be able to calculate the correct quantity of medication to be dispensed based on the prescribed dose and days supply.
- Concentration: This refers to the quantity of a drug present in a specific volume or weight of a solution. Pharmacy technicians need to be able to accurately calculate the concentration of medication to compound and dispense it properly.

Equipment and supplies required for drug administration.

Package Size

The type of equipment and supplies needed for administering drugs can differ based on the medication type and its method of administration. However, some standard items are typically used across various medications. These include:

- Syringes: These are used for accurately measuring and administering medication. They come in various sizes and can be for oral or injectable use.
- Needles: These are used for piercing the skin and delivering medication into the body. They come in different sizes, depending on the administration method and the medication being given.
- IV bags and tubing: These are used for intravenous medications. IV bags are sterile containers that hold the medication and are connected to the patient via tubing inserted into a vein.
- Inhalers: These devices deliver medication directly into the lungs. They come in different types, such as metered-dose inhalers and dry powder inhalers.
- Topical applicators: Items like cotton swabs or sterile gauze are used to apply medication to the skin.
- Enteral feeding tubes: These tubes deliver medication directly into the stomach or intestines. They come in different sizes and can be either nasogastric or gastrostomy tubes.

When preparing for drug administration, it's crucial to ensure all equipment and supplies are correctly labeled, clean, and sterile to avoid contamination and ensure patient safety. Also, the right package size of the medication should be chosen based on the prescribed dose and administration method.

Unit Dose

Unit dose dispensing is a common drug distribution method that involves dispensing medications in pre-packaged, single-dose units. This method improves accuracy, safety, and efficiency in medication administration.

Several pieces of equipment and supplies are needed for unit dose dispensing, including:

- Automated dispensing cabinets (ADCs): These allow for the secure storage and dispensing of medications in pre-packaged doses. ADCs are commonly used in hospitals and other healthcare facilities to improve medication safety and efficiency.

- Unit dose packaging materials: These may include pre-packaged medication blister packs, pouches, or syringes. These materials package individual doses of medications for dispensing to patients.

- Barcode scanners: These scan the medication packaging to ensure accuracy in dispensing and administration.

- Labels: These are used to identify each medication, its dose, and any necessary patient information such as name and room number.

- Medication carts: These are used to transport pre-packaged doses of medication from the pharmacy to the patient care unit.

Pharmacy technicians should be familiar with the equipment and supplies needed for unit dose dispensing and the procedures for dispensing and administering medications in this way.

Diabetic Supplies

Diabetes is a condition where the body can't properly process glucose, leading to high blood sugar levels. Diabetic individuals may require insulin injections and/or additional drugs, as well as supplies for glucose monitoring and insulin administration, in addition to their prescribed medication.

Here are some standard diabetic supplies that may be needed for drug administration:

1. Insulin syringes: These small needles inject insulin into the body. They come in different sizes and gauges, and patients must choose the appropriate size for their needs.

2. Insulin pens: These pre-filled pens contain insulin, which patients can use to inject insulin into their bodies. The pen has a dial that allows the patient to set the correct dose.

3. Glucometers: These devices are used to monitor blood sugar levels. Patients prick their fingers to get a small blood sample, which is then placed on a test strip and inserted into the glucometer for analysis. This helps the patient determine if their blood sugar levels are within the desired range.

4. Lancets: These small needles are used to prick the finger to get a blood sample for use with a glucometer.

5. Test strips: These small strips are used to test the blood sugar levels on the glucometer.

6. Alcohol swabs: These are used to clean the injection site before administering insulin and the skin before getting a blood sample.

By understanding the various types of diabetic supplies needed for drug administration, pharmacy technicians can ensure patients receive the correct supplies and use them properly. Pharmacy technicians should be familiar with these supplies to provide accurate patient information and answer questions.

Spacers

Individuals suffering from respiratory disorders such as asthma or Chronic Obstructive Pulmonary Disease (COPD) must use spacers when inhaling medication. A spacer is an auxiliary chamber that can be affixed to an inhaler to enhance the delivery of medication to the lungs.

To administer medication with a spacer, you need the following tools and supplies:

- Inhaler: This device dispenses the medication to the patient.
- Spacer: This is the chamber that is connected to the inhaler's end.
- Mouthpiece: This component of the spacer is used by the patient to inhale the medication.
- Mask: Some spacers come with a mask attachment, which can be used for patients who have difficulty using a mouthpiece.

It's crucial to ensure that the spacer is suitable for the patient, as they come in different sizes to accommodate different ages and lung capacities. Additionally, spacers should be cleaned regularly to avoid the accumulation of medication residue or bacteria.

Pharmacy technicians can help ensure that medications are administered effectively and safely by providing patients with the appropriate tools and supplies.

Oral Medication

Oral medication administration is a common method of drug delivery. The following equipment and supplies are needed for oral medication administration:

- Dosage forms: These can be tablets, capsules, liquids, powders, and more.
- Measuring devices: These are used to accurately measure the amount of medication being administered. They include oral syringes, droppers, and spoons.
- Cups: These are used to safely and conveniently administer liquid medications.
- Pill crushers: These are used to crush pills into a fine powder for easier swallowing.
- Water: This is used to help swallow the medication and ensure it reaches the stomach.

When administering oral medications, it's important to confirm the patient's identity, the medication being administered, and the dosage. Additionally, it's crucial to ensure that the patient can swallow the medication and check for any potential drug interactions or contraindications.

Injectable Syringes

Injectable medications are a common method of drug administration, and the correct equipment and supplies are essential for safe and effective medication delivery. Injectable medications can be administered subcutaneously, intramuscularly, or intravenously, and the type of syringe and needle used will depend on the specific route of administration.

Syringes are available in various sizes, the most common being 1 mL, 3 mL, and 5 mL. The size of the syringe is determined by the volume of medication that needs to be administered. The more potent the medication, the larger the syringe should be. For instance, a medication that requires 1 mL to be administered should be given using a 1 mL syringe.

In addition to the syringe's size, the type of needle used is also important. Needles come in various lengths and gauges, with the needle's length depending on the depth of the injection site. The gauge of the needle refers to the thickness of the needle, with a higher gauge number indicating a thinner needle. Thinner needles are typically used for more viscous medications, as they can be easier to administer.

Other supplies needed for injectable medication administration include alcohol swabs, gauze pads, and a sharps container for safe needle disposal. Pharmacy technicians must ensure that they have all necessary supplies on hand and are using them correctly to ensure patient safety.

Lot numbers, expiration dates, and National Drug Code (NDC) numbers

The inclusion of expiration dates, lot numbers, and National Drug Code (NDC) numbers is crucial in drug orders and prescriptions. A lot number is a unique code given by the manufacturer to a specific batch of medication. This code is significant in case there is a need for a recall or if an issue arises with the medication.

The expiration date is also of great importance as it shows when the medication is no longer safe or effective. Pharmacy technicians need to meticulously check these dates and ensure that no medication is dispensed past its expiration date.

The National Drug Code (NDC) is a 10-digit code that encapsulates the identity, dosage strength, and unit of packaging of a medication. It is utilized by pharmacies, insurance companies, and other healthcare providers for tracking and managing the use of medication. Pharmacy technicians need to be well-acquainted with the NDC numbering system and make sure it is included in all drug orders and prescriptions.

For the safety and efficiency of the pharmacy, it is vital to correctly identify and manage dispensable, non-dispensable, and expired medications and supplies. Pharmacy technicians can contribute to this by knowing where to find these items and how to properly return them.

Dispensable medications and supplies are those that have been dispensed to a patient but are no longer needed. These items should be properly identified, recorded, and returned to stock if they are in good condition and have not expired. If the item has been opened or partially used, it should be discarded.

Non-dispensable medications and supplies are those that are received but not meant for dispensing, such as samples or clinical trial supplies. These items should be properly identified and stored separately from dispensable items.

Expired medications and supplies should be identified and removed from the pharmacy inventory. Depending on the pharmacy's policy and procedure, these items may be returned to the manufacturer or distributor for credit, returned to stock for destruction, or sent to a reverse distributor for proper disposal.

Returning expired or unusable medications to the manufacturer or distributor in exchange for credit is known as credit return. These items should be properly packaged and labeled with the necessary documentation, including the expiration date, lot number, and National Drug Code (NDC) number.

Stock return involves returning unopened, non-expired medications and supplies to the pharmacy inventory for future use. These items should be properly labeled with the necessary documentation and stored in the appropriate location.

Reverse distribution is the process of returning expired medications to a reverse distributor for proper disposal. Reverse distributors are licensed and regulated entities that specialize in properly handling and disposing of expired medications. Pharmacy technicians must be familiar with the correct procedures for preparing and labeling items for return to a reverse distributor.

Chapter 8: Practice Test

1. Essential Exam Topics and Concepts

"This segment delves into a broad spectrum of pharmaceutical theories and practices. It's crucial to have a comprehensive understanding of these subjects as they lay the groundwork for the expertise of a pharmacy technician."

1.1 What does pharmacokinetics aim to study?

a) The interaction between drugs

b) The impact of drugs on the body

c) The absorption, distribution, metabolism, and excretion of drugs

d) The interaction of drugs with other drugs

1.1 Answer: c) The absorption, distribution, metabolism, and excretion of drugs.

1.2 What is the main role of an antagonist drug?

a) To amplify the effect of another drug

b) To inhibit or minimize the effect of another drug

c) To treat bacterial infections

d) To alleviate pain and inflammation

1.2 Answer: b) To inhibit or minimize the effect of another drug.

1.3 How would you define pharmacodynamics?

a) The study of drug movement within the body

b) The study of drug absorption into the bloodstream

c) The study of drug interaction with specific drug receptors

d) The study of drug elimination from the body

1.3 Answer: c) The study of drug interaction with specific drug receptors.

1.4 Which drug dosage form does not go through the digestive system?

a) Oral tablets

b) Intravenous injections

c) Sublingual tablets

d) Transdermal patches

1.4 Answer: b) Intravenous injections.

1.5 Which drug schedule category is most prone to abuse?

a) Schedule I

b) Schedule II

c) Schedule III

d) Schedule IV

1.5 Answer: a) Schedule I.

1.6 What does "pharmacology" mean?

a) The study of drugs and their effects on living organisms

b) The study of the physical and chemical properties of drugs

c) The study of drug synthesis in the laboratory

d) The study of drug prescription and dispensing to patients

1.6 Answer: a) The study of drugs and their effects on living organisms.

1.7 What is the main responsibility of a pharmaceutics pharmacist?

a) To create new drug formulations

b) To dispense medications to patients

c) To oversee patients' medication therapy

d) To educate patients on medication usage

1.7 Answer: a) To create new drug formulations.

1.8 Can you give an example of a controlled substance?

a) Aspirin

b) Insulin

c) Ibuprofen

d) Oxycodone

1.8 Answer: d) Oxycodone.

1.9 Why are drug recalls necessary?

a) To guarantee the safety and efficacy of drugs in the market

b) To monitor drug prices and availability

c) To regulate drug advertising and promotion

d) To track adverse drug reactions in patients

1.9 Answer: a) To guarantee the safety and efficacy of drugs in the market.

1.10 Which federal agency oversees pharmacy compounding practices?

a) Drug Enforcement Administration (DEA)

b) Food and Drug Administration (FDA)

c) Centers for Disease Control and Prevention (CDC)

d) National Institutes of Health (NIH)

1.10 Answer: b) Food and Drug Administration (FDA).

1.11 Which organ primarily metabolizes drugs?

a) Kidneys

b) Liver

c) Lungs

d) Pancreas

1.11 Answer: b) Liver.

1.12 How would you define bioavailability?

a) The rate at which a drug is eliminated from the body

b) The process of drug absorption into the bloodstream

c) The portion of a drug that reaches systemic circulation unchanged

d) The time it takes for a drug to produce its therapeutic effect

1.12 Answer: c) The portion of a drug that reaches systemic circulation unchanged.

1.13 Which drug administration route has the quickest onset of action?

a) Oral

b) Subcutaneous

c) Intravenous

d) Transdermal

1.13 Answer: c) Intravenous.

1.14 What is the main aim of a drug formulary?

a) To list all available medications in a pharmacy

b) To provide information on drug interactions

c) To ensure appropriate medication usage and cost-effective therapy

d) To monitor medication errors in healthcare settings

1.14 Answer: c) To ensure appropriate medication usage and cost-effective therapy.

1.15 Which drug reference would you use to identify a drug's adverse effects?

a) Package insert

b) Drug monograph

c) Pharmacopeia

d) Drug interaction checker

1.15 Answer: a) Package insert.

1.16 What is the action mechanism of a beta-blocker medication?

a) Vasodilation

b) Increase heart rate

c) Inhibit activity of the sympathetic nervous system

d) Enhance blood clotting

1.16 Answer: c) Inhibit activity of the sympathetic nervous system.

1.17 What is the main function of an ACE inhibitor medication?

a) Lower blood pressure

b) Reduce cholesterol levels

c) Increase insulin sensitivity

d) Relieve pain and inflammation

1.17 Answer: a) Lower blood pressure.

1.18 Which of the following drugs is classified as an anticoagulant?

a) Metformin

b) Warfarin

c) Metoprolol

d) Levothyroxine

1.18 Answer: b) Warfarin.

1.19 What is the aim of medication reconciliation?

a) To ensure accurate medication billing

b) To monitor patients' adherence to medication therapy

c) To compare a patient's current medication list with the most recent prescription

d) To identify potential drug-drug interactions

1.19 Answer: c) To compare a patient's current medication list with the most recent prescription.

1.20 Which drug classification is typically used to treat high blood pressure?

a) Antihistamines

b) Diuretics

c) Antibiotics

d) Antidepressants

1.20 Answer: b) Diuretics.

2. Pharmaceutical Calculations

For pharmacy technicians, it's essential to have a strong grasp of calculation techniques and formulas. Multiple-choice questions in this area might test your ability to accurately execute dosage calculations and compounding.

2.1 What's the right formula to calculate the flow rate for an intravenous infusion?

a) Flow rate (mL/h) = Volume (mL) / Time (hours)

b) Flow rate (mL/min) = Volume (mL) / Time (minutes)

c) Flow rate (mL/h) = Time (hours) / Volume (mL)

d) Flow rate (mL/min) = Time (minutes) / Volume (mL)

2.1 Answer: a) Flow rate (mL/h) = Volume (mL) / Time (hours).

2.2 If a prescription requires 500 mg of medication to be taken orally and the medication is available in 250 mg tablets, how many tablets should be given?

a) 2 tablets

b) 1 tablet

c) 3 tablets

d) 4 tablets

2.2 Answer: a) 2 tablets.

2.3 How many milliliters make up 1 teaspoon?

a) 2 mL

b) 5 mL

c) 10 mL

d) 15 mL

2.3 Answer: c) 10 mL.

2.4 If a medication is ordered to be administered at 60 drops per minute and the drop factor is 15 gtt/mL, what should the flow rate be in mL/hour?

a) 4 mL/hour

b) 15 mL/hour

c) 30 mL/hour

d) 60 mL/hour

2.4 Answer: b) 15 mL/hour.

2.5 If a patient needs to take 0.25 mg of a medication and the available tablets are 0.5 mg each, how many tablets should the patient take?

a) 1 tablet

b) 2 tablets

c) 0.5 tablets

d) 0.25 tablets

2.5 Answer: a) 1 tablet.

2.6 If a medication contains 250 mg of active ingredient in 5 mL of solution, what is the ratio strength?

a) 50 mg/mL

b) 25 mg/mL

c) 5 mg/mL

d) 0.25 mg/mL

2.6 Answer: b) 25 mg/mL.

2.7 How many milliliters are there in 1 fluid ounce?

a) 30 mL

b) 15 mL

c) 10 mL

d) 5 mL

2.7 Answer: a) 30 mL.

2.8 If a patient is prescribed 40 mg of medication to be taken four times daily for seven days, what's the total milligrams of medication that should be dispensed?

a) 80 mg

b) 160 mg

c) 280 mg

d) 1120 mg

2.8 Answer: d) 1120 mg.

2.9 If a pharmacist needs to compound a 2% w/v solution of a medication using a 500 mL solvent, how many grams of the medication should be added?

a) 1 g

b) 5 g

c) 10 g

d) 20 g

2.9 Answer: b) 5 g.

2.10 How many milligrams are in 1 gram?

a) 100 mg

b) 500 mg

c) 1000 mg

d) 5000 mg

2.10 Answer: c) 1000 mg.

2.11 If a medication is ordered to be administered at a rate of 0.5 mg/kg/day and the patient weighs 70 kg, how many milligrams of medication should be administered in a 24-hour period?

a) 25 mg

b) 35 mg

c) 50 mg

d) 70 mg

2.11 Answer: b) 35 mg.

2.12 If a prescription calls for administering 2 teaspoons of medication every 4 hours, how many milliliters of medication should be administered in a 24-hour period?

a) 12 mL

b) 24 mL

c) 48 mL

d) 96 mL

2.12 Answer: c) 48 mL.

2.13 What's the right formula to calculate the body mass index (BMI)?

a) BMI = Weight (kg) × Height (cm)

b) BMI = Weight (kg) / Height (m^2)

c) BMI = Weight (lb) × Height (in)

d) BMI = Weight (lb) / Height (ft^2)

2.13 Answer: b) BMI = Weight (kg) / Height (m^2).

2.14 If a medication is ordered to be administered at a rate of 5 mcg/kg/minute, the patient weighs 60 kg, and the medication is available as a 500 mcg/mL solution, what should be the flow rate in mL/hour?

a) 10 mL/hour

b) 20 mL/hour

c) 30 mL/hour

d) 40 mL/hour

2.14 Answer: c) 30 mL/hour.

2.15 How many milliliters of a 10% w/v solution can be made from 15 grams of active ingredient?

a) 150 mL

b) 100 mL

c) 50 mL

d) 15 mL

2.15 Answer: a) 150 mL.

2.16 If a patient is prescribed 0.125 mg of a medication and the available tablets are 0.25 mg each, how many tablets should the patient take?

a) 1 tablet

b) 2 tablets

c) 0.5 tablets

d) 0.25 tablets

2.16 Answer: b) 2 tablets.

2.17 What's the right formula to calculate the body surface area (BSA) using the Mosteller formula?

a) BSA = (Height [cm] × Weight [kg]) / 3600

b) BSA = (Height [cm] × Weight [kg]) / 3131

c) BSA = (Height [m] × Weight [kg]) / 3600

d) BSA = (Height [m] × Weight [kg]) / 3131

2.17 Answer: b) BSA = (Height [cm] × Weight [kg]) / 3131.

2.18 If a medication is ordered to be administered at a rate of 10 mcg/min and the medication is available as a 0.1 mg/mL solution, what should be the flow rate in mL/hour?

a) 0.6 mL/hour

b) 1 mL/hour

c) 6 mL/hour

d) 10 mL/hour

2.18 Answer: a) 0.6 mL/hour.

2.19 What's the right formula to calculate the creatinine clearance using the Cockcroft-Gault formula?

a) Creatinine clearance (mL/min) = (140 - Age) / (Scr × Weight)

b) Creatinine clearance (mL/min) = (140 - Age) / (Scr × Weight) × 0.85

c) Creatinine clearance (mL/min) = (140 - Age) × (Scr × Weight)

d) Creatinine clearance (mL/min) = (140 - Age) × (Scr × Weight) × 0.85

2.19 Answer: b) Creatinine clearance (mL/min) = (140 - Age) / (Scr × Weight) × 0.85.

2.20 If a medication is available as 125 mg/5 mL, how many milliliters should be given to administer 500 mg of the medication?

a) 10 mL

b) 15 mL

c) 20 mL

d) 25 mL

2.20 Answer: d) 25 mL.

3. Understanding Drug Categories and Terms

"Multiple choice questions in this section will assess your knowledge of various drug categories, their roles, and the related terminology. Understanding drug categories and terms is crucial for safe and efficient medication administration."

3.1 Which of the following drug categories is typically used for hypertension treatment?

a) NSAIDs

b) Anticoagulants

c) Antihistamines

d) Antihypertensives

3.1 Answer: d) Antihypertensives.

3.2 What term is used to describe a drug's capacity to alleviate pain without causing unconsciousness?

a) Analgesic

b) Anesthetic

c) Antipyretic

d) Anticoagulant

3.2 Answer: a) Analgesic.

3.3 Which drug category is used for treating bacterial infections?

a) Antidepressants

b) Antidiabetics

c) Antibiotics

d) Antipsychotics

3.3 Answer: c) Antibiotics.

3.4 Which drug category is used to decrease blood glucose levels in diabetes patients?

a) Anticoagulants

b) Antihypertensives

c) Antilipemics

d) Antidiabetics

3.4 Answer: d) Antidiabetics.

3.5 Which drug category is used to lessen inflammation and alleviate pain?

a) Anticoagulants

b) Anticonvulsants

c) Antidiarrheals

d) Nonsteroidal anti-inflammatory drugs (NSAIDs)

3.5 Answer: d) Nonsteroidal anti-inflammatory drugs (NSAIDs).

3.6 What term is used to describe a drug's ability to inhibit or prevent microorganism growth?

a) Antipyretic

b) Antiseptic

c) Antitussive

d) Antibiotic

3.6 Answer: d) Antibiotic.

3.7 Which drug category is used to treat allergies and allergic reactions?

a) Antidiabetics

b) Antihistamines

c) Antipsychotics

d) Antihypertensives

3.7 Answer: b) Antihistamines.

3.8 What term is used to describe a drug's ability to induce sleep or promote sedation?

a) Analgesic

b) Anesthetic

c) Antipyretic

d) Hypnotic

3.8 Answer: d) Hypnotic.

3.9 Which drug category is used to prevent the formation of blood clots?

a) Anticoagulants

b) Antidiarrheals

c) Antihistamines

d) Antivirals

3.9 Answer: a) Anticoagulants.

3.10 Which of the following drug categories is typically used to treat depression and anxiety disorders?

a) Antidepressants

b) Antihypertensives

c) Anticonvulsants

d) Antidiabetics

3.10 Answer: a) Antidepressants.

4. Pharmacy Legislation and Guidelines

"This section will likely include questions about federal and state laws that regulate pharmacy practice. It's crucial for pharmacy technicians to understand these laws and adhere to them to ensure patient safety and regulatory compliance."

4.1 Who is the federal authority responsible for approving and regulating prescription drugs in the United States?

a) Food and Drug Administration (FDA)

b) Drug Enforcement Administration (DEA)

c) Centers for Medicare and Medicaid Services (CMS)

d) Occupational Safety and Health Administration (OSHA)

4.1 Answer: a) Food and Drug Administration (FDA).

4.2 Which law mandates that prescription medications be dispensed in containers that are resistant to child access?

a) Drug Approval Modernization Act

b) Controlled Substances Act

c) Poison Prevention Packaging Act

d) Affordable Care Act

4.2 Answer: c) Poison Prevention Packaging Act.

4.3 Which federal legislation prohibits the unauthorized disclosure of patient health data and sets privacy standards?

a) Food, Drug, and Cosmetic Act

b) Drug Quality and Security Act

c) Health Insurance Portability and Accountability Act (HIPAA)

d) Americans with Disabilities Act (ADA)

4.3 Answer: c) Health Insurance Portability and Accountability Act (HIPAA).

4.4 What term is used to describe the process of checking the accuracy and completeness of a prescription before dispensing the medication?

a) Prescription transcription

b) Prescription validation

c) Prescription dispensing

d) Prescription verification

4.4 Answer: d) Prescription verification.

4.5 Which federal law mandates that pharmacies keep patient records for a minimum of ___ years?

a) 1

b) 3

c) 5

d) 7

4.5 Answer: d) 7.

4.6 Which agency oversees the regulation of handling and disposal of hazardous substances in the workplace?

a) Drug Enforcement Administration (DEA)

b) Food and Drug Administration (FDA)

c) Occupational Safety and Health Administration (OSHA)

d) Drug Enforcement Agency (DEA)

4.6 Answer: c) Occupational Safety and Health Administration (OSHA).

4.7 Which law regulates the sale and distribution of controlled substances?

a) Drug Approval Modernization Act

b) Poison Prevention Packaging Act

c) Controlled Substances Act

d) Health Insurance Portability and Accountability Act (HIPAA)

4.7 Answer: c) Controlled Substances Act.

4.8 What term is used to describe the process of moving a prescription from one pharmacy to another?

a) Prescription filling

b) Prescription compounding

c) Prescription dispensing

d) Prescription transfer

4.8 Answer: d) Prescription transfer.

4.9 Which federal law mandates that pharmacies offer patient counseling for new prescription medications?

a) Food, Drug, and Cosmetic Act

b) Drug Quality and Security Act

c) Health Insurance Portability and Accountability Act (HIPAA)

d) Omnibus Budget Reconciliation Act (OBRA)

4.9 Answer: d) Omnibus Budget Reconciliation Act (OBRA).

4.10 Can you give an example of a Schedule II controlled substance?

a) Acetaminophen with codeine

b) Lorazepam

c) Diphenhydramine

d) Montelukast

4.10 Answer: a) Acetaminophen with codeine.

5. Medication Order Entry and Processing

"This section may test your understanding of reading prescriptions, dispensing medications, and reconciling medications. The tasks require a keen eye for detail and accuracy, which are essential skills for a pharmacy technician."

5.1 What term is used to describe the process of reading a prescription and inputting the medication order into the pharmacy system?

a) Medication reconciliation

b) Medication therapy management

c) Prescription dispensing

d) Prescription interpretation

5.1 Answer: d) Prescription interpretation.

5.2 Which U.S. federal law mandates that prescriptions for controlled substances be sent electronically to the pharmacy?

a) Controlled Substances Act

b) Poison Prevention Packaging Act

c) Drug Quality and Security Act

d) Drug Approval Modernization Act

5.2 Answer: c) Drug Quality and Security Act.

5.3 What term is used to describe the verification of the correctness and completeness of a medication order before the medication is dispensed?

a) Medication reconciliation

b) Medication therapy management

c) Medication validation

d) Medication dispensing

5.3 Answer: c) Medication validation.

5.4 What abbreviation is used on a prescription to mean "as needed"?

a) PRN

b) QID

c) QD

d) BID

5.4 Answer: a) PRN.

5.5 What term is used to describe the process of preparing a medication specifically for a patient based on a prescription?

a) Medication reconciliation

b) Medication therapy management

c) Medication compounding

d) Medication dispensing

5.5 Answer: c) Medication compounding.

5.6 Which U.S. federal agency supervises the Drug Enforcement Administration (DEA) registration process for pharmacies?

a) Food and Drug Administration (FDA)

b) Drug Enforcement Administration (DEA)

c) Occupational Safety and Health Administration (OSHA)

d) Centers for Medicare and Medicaid Services (CMS)

5.6 Answer: a) Food and Drug Administration (FDA).

5.7 What term is used to describe the process of comparing a patient's current list of medications with a newly prescribed medication to identify any inconsistencies or potential interactions?

a) Medication reconciliation

b) Medication therapy management

c) Medication evaluation

d) Medication dispensing

5.7 Answer: a) Medication reconciliation.

5.8 What abbreviation is used on a prescription to mean "twice a day"?

a) BID

b) TID

c) QID

d) PRN

5.8 Answer: a) BID.

5.9 Which U.S. federal law requires pharmacies to keep records of dispensed medications for a certain period of time?

a) Controlled Substances Act

b) Poison Prevention Packaging Act

c) Health Insurance Portability and Accountability Act (HIPAA)

d) Omnibus Budget Reconciliation Act (OBRA)

5.9 Answer: d) Omnibus Budget Reconciliation Act (OBRA).

5.10 What term is used to describe the process of delivering a medication to a patient's specified location?

a) Medication reconciliation

b) Medication therapy management

c) Medication distribution

d) Medication dispensing

5.10 Answer: c) Medication distribution.

6. Ensuring Medication Safety and Quality

"Because medication safety is of utmost importance, you should anticipate multiple-choice questions that evaluate your comprehension of the optimal methods for dispensing, storing, and avoiding medication errors. It's crucial to understand quality assurance procedures to uphold patient safety."

6.1 Which entity is in charge of accrediting healthcare institutions and advocating for medication safety?

a) Food and Drug Administration (FDA)

b) Centers for Disease Control and Prevention (CDC)

c) Institute for Safe Medication Practices (ISMP)

d) Drug Enforcement Administration (DEA)

6.1 Answer: c) Institute for Safe Medication Practices (ISMP).

6.2 What does the "beyond-use date" on a medication label signify?

a) It shows the medication's expiration date

b) It ensures the medication is stored correctly

c) It identifies the patient's specific medication dosage

d) It records the medication's lot number for quality control

6.2 Answer: a) It shows the medication's expiration date.

6.3 What is the correct storage condition for a medication that needs refrigeration?

a) Stored at room temperature

b) Exposed to direct sunlight

c) Stored in the freezer

d) Stored in a high humidity environment

6.3 Answer: c) Stored in the refrigerator.

6.4 What is the main function of a medication barcode scanning system?

a) To monitor medication inventory levels

b) To ensure precise medication dispensing

c) To track patient medication adherence

d) To aid with medication compounding

6.4 Answer: b) To ensure precise medication dispensing.

6.5 What term is used to describe the process of checking and confirming medication orders for accuracy and suitability?

a) Medication reconciliation

b) Medication verification

c) Medication compounding

d) Medication transcription

6.5 Answer: b) Medication verification.

6.6 In the context of medication safety, what does the acronym "MAR" represent?

a) Medication Administration Record

b) Medication Authorization Request

c) Medication Assessment Report

d) Medication Adherence Review

6.6 Answer: a) Medication Administration Record.

6.7 What factor leads to medication errors resulting from medications that look or sound similar?

a) Insufficient storage conditions

b) Poor medication labeling

c) High medication dosage

d) Similar drug names or packaging

6.7 Answer: d) Similar drug names or packaging.

6.8 What is the main purpose of a medication safety data sheet (MSDS)?

a) To provide information on potential medication side effects

b) To detail proper medication administration techniques

c) To ensure correct disposal methods for unused medications

d) To provide safety information for handling hazardous medications

6.8 Answer: d) To provide safety information for handling hazardous medications.

6.9 In the context of medication safety, what does the acronym "CPOE" represent?

a) Controlled Prescription Order Entry

b) Centralized Patient Order Entry

c) Computerized Physician Order Entry

d) Coordinated Prescription Order Enforcement

6.9 Answer: c) Computerized Physician Order Entry.

6.10 Which procedure involves checking the medication label against the medication order before dispensing?

a) Medication reconciliation

b) Medication compounding

c) Medication verification

d) Medication dispensing

6.10 Answer: c) Medication verification.

7. Pharmacy Inventory Management

This section may contain multiple-choice questions about inventory control, purchasing processes, and managing drug expiry dates. It's important for pharmacy technicians to know how to keep inventory at the right levels and ensure the availability of medications.

7.1 What inventory management method is used to keep inventory levels in line with patient demand while reducing carrying costs?

a) FIFO (First-In, First-Out)

b) LIFO (Last-In, First-Out)

c) JIT (Just-in-Time)

d) ABC (Always Better Control)

7.1 Answer: c) JIT (Just-in-Time).

7.2 In pharmacy inventory management, what does "par level" mean?

a) The minimum amount of a medication that should always be in stock

b) The maximum amount of a medication that can be ordered at once

c) The daily average quantity of a medication used

d) The total value of medications in the pharmacy inventory

7.2 Answer: a) The minimum amount of a medication that should always be in stock.

7.3 Why are regular medication inventory audits conducted in a pharmacy?

a) To identify medications that have expired or are about to expire for disposal

b) To find out the total value of medications in stock

c) To monitor the accuracy of medication dispensing by comparing inventory records

d) To ensure adherence to medication storage guidelines

7.3 Answer: a) To identify medications that have expired or are about to expire for disposal.

7.4 Which inventory management technique helps to avoid stock shortages and ensures timely availability of medications?

a) Consignment inventory

b) Economic order quantity (EOQ)

c) Stock rotation

d) Vendor-managed inventory (VMI)

7.4 Answer: d) Vendor-managed inventory (VMI).

7.5 Why is a perpetual inventory system used in a pharmacy?

a) To track medication prices and calculate profit margins

b) To keep inventory records accurate and current

c) To automate the process of dispensing medications

d) To create medication usage reports for regulatory purposes

7.5 Answer: b) To keep inventory records accurate and current.

7.6 What should be taken into account when deciding when to reorder medications in pharmacy inventory management?

a) The demand for the medication from patients

b) The expiration date of the medication

c) The fluctuation in the price of the medication

d) The storage requirements of the medication

7.6 Answer: a) The demand for the medication from patients.

7.7 Why is a medication return policy implemented in a pharmacy?

a) To discourage patients from returning medications for refunds

b) To ensure the disposal of expired or recalled medications

c) To lower medication costs by reusing returned medications

d) To comply with regulations regarding medication returns

7.7 Answer: b) To ensure the disposal of expired or recalled medications.

7.8 Which inventory management method prioritizes medications based on their usage value?

a) Stock rotation

b) ABC analysis

c) Par level ordering

d) Just-in-Time (JIT) inventory

7.8 Answer: b) ABC analysis.

7.9 What practice can help avoid wasting medications due to expiration or non-use?

a) Storing medications in a warm and humid environment

b) Dispensing larger amounts of medications to patients

c) Counseling patients on medication use to ensure proper usage

d) Using appropriate medication storage and rotation techniques

7.9 Answer: d) Using appropriate medication storage and rotation techniques.

7.10 Why is a barcode scanning system used for medication inventory management?

a) To track medication prices for pricing adjustments

b) To automate the medication ordering process

c) To enhance the accuracy of medication dispensing and minimize errors

d) To create financial reports for inventory valuation

7.10 Answer: c) To enhance the accuracy of medication dispensing and minimize errors.

8. Pharmacy Information Systems

"This section may contain questions about pharmacy software, electronic health records, and the role of technology in pharmacy practice. It's crucial to understand pharmacy information systems to ensure a smooth workflow and accurate documentation."

8.1 Can you give an example of a pharmacy information system?

a) Barcode scanner

b) Prescription label printer

c) Medication dispensing robot

d) Prescription vial

8.1 Answer: c) Medication dispensing robot.

8.2 What is the main function of electronic health records (EHRs) in pharmacy practice?

a) Monitoring medication inventory levels

b) Facilitating communication with healthcare providers

c) Automating medication dispensing processes

d) Managing patient medication profiles

8.2 Answer: d) To manage patient medication profiles.

8.3 What role does pharmacy software play in medication dispensing?

a) Ensuring patient privacy and data security

b) Tracking prescription refill requests

c) Generating medication labels for dispensing

d) Calculating medication dosages

8.3 Answer: c) To generate medication labels for dispensing.

8.4 How can pharmacy information systems enhance medication safety?

a) By automating medication compounding processes

b) By providing drug interaction alerts and allergy checks

c) By monitoring pharmacy staff productivity

d) By reducing medication dispensing costs

8.4 Answer: b) By providing drug interaction alerts and allergy checks.

8.5 What is an advantage of using barcode scanning technology in pharmacy practice?

a) Better medication storage organization

b) Increased patient medication adherence

c) Improved medication compounding accuracy

d) Lowered medication reimbursement rates

8.5 Answer: c) Enhanced medication compounding accuracy.

8.6 What is the aim of electronic prescribing (e-prescribing) systems in pharmacy practice?

a) Automating medication ordering from suppliers

b) Streamlining the medication dispensing process

c) Providing electronic signature capabilities for prescriptions

d) Tracking medication expiration dates

8.6 Answer: b) To streamline the medication dispensing process.

8.7 What is a feature of a strong pharmacy inventory management system?

a) Automatic medication dispensing capabilities

b) Real-time tracking of medication deliveries

c) Integration with patient billing systems

d) Monthly inventory stock reporting

8.7 Answer: b) Real-time tracking of medication deliveries.

8.8 What is the main advantage of using automated medication dispensing systems in a pharmacy?

a) Fewer medication dispensing errors

b) Reduced medication storage capacity

c) Enhanced patient counseling services

d) More efficient medication procurement processes

8.8 Answer: a) Reduced medication dispensing errors.

8.9 How can pharmacy information systems aid patient counseling services?

a) By producing medication instructions and educational materials

b) By improving communication with healthcare providers

c) By automating medication dispensing processes

d) By monitoring patient medication adherence rates

8.9 Answer: a) By generating medication instructions and educational materials.

8.10 What is the function of a pharmacy management system?

a) Monitoring pharmacy staff productivity

b) Automating medication ordering processes

c) Providing real-time inventory stock tracking

d) Calculating medication dispensing costs

8.10 Answer: c) To provide real-time inventory stock tracking.

9. Understanding Medication Adherence and Patient Education

"Multiple-choice questions in this section will evaluate your grasp of methods to encourage medication adherence and educate patients. Recognizing the significance of medication adherence and effective patient communication is crucial."

9.1 What is the main objective of medication adherence?

a) To lower the chance of adverse drug reactions.

b) To cut down on healthcare expenses.

c) To ensure accurate documentation of medication.

d) To enhance patient satisfaction.

9.1 Answer: a) To lower the chance of adverse drug reactions.

9.2 What factors can lead to non-adherence to medication?

a) Complicated medication schedules.

b) Sufficient patient education.

c) Regular reminders for refilling medication.

d) Supportive healthcare provider.

9.2 Answer: a) Complicated medication schedules.

9.3 What is the role of a pharmacy technician in encouraging medication adherence?

a) Timely dispensing of medications.

b) Providing patients with accurate medication information.

c) Monitoring rates of patient adherence.

d) Evaluating medication side effects.

9.3 Answer: b) Providing patients with accurate medication information.

9.4 What communication technique is most effective in improving patient medication adherence?

a) Using medical terms to explain medication instructions.

b) Providing only written instructions.

c) Engaging in active listening and providing clear explanations.

d) Solely relying on electronic reminders.

9.4 Answer: c) Engaging in active listening and providing clear explanations.

9.5 What strategies can address medication affordability issues for patients?

a) Recommending alternatives available over-the-counter.

b) Exploring patient assistance programs.

c) Encouraging the substitution of generic medication.

d) Increasing the dosage of medication.

9.5 Answer: b) Exploring patient assistance programs.

9.6 How can pharmacy technicians aid in educating patients?

a) Conducting sessions on medication therapy management (MTM).

b) Administering surveys on patient satisfaction.

c) Providing reminders for medication refills.

d) Assisting with reconciling medications.

9.6 Answer: a) Conducting sessions on medication therapy management (MTM).

9.7 Which of the following is an example of a health literacy barrier to medication adherence?

a) Proficiency in language of the patient.

b) Clear instructions for medication.

c) Low cost of medication.

d) Adequate healthcare coverage.

9.7 Answer: a) Proficiency in language of the patient.

9.8 What is the main purpose of counseling patients about medication?

a) To ensure proper storage of medication.

b) To address potential interactions between drugs.

c) To monitor rates of medication adherence.

d) To encourage patient involvement in healthcare decisions.

9.8 Answer: b) To address potential interactions between drugs.

9.9 How can pharmacy technicians help patients manage medication side effects?

a) Recommending supplements available over-the-counter.

b) Monitoring patient compliance with medication.

c) Educating about expected side effects.

d) Adjusting dosages of medication without consultation.

9.9 Answer: c) Educating about expected side effects.

9.10 Which of the following interventions is most effective in improving medication adherence?

a) Educating patients about the importance of adherence.

b) Use of complex medication packaging.

c) Frequent changes in medication formulations.

d) Minimal involvement of patients in healthcare decisions.

9.10 Answer: a) Educating patients about the importance of adherence.

10. Mixing and Sterile Formulations

"This segment may contain multiple-choice questions about the techniques of mixing, aseptic procedures, and the management of sterile formulations. The ability to demonstrate an understanding of the principles of mixing and maintaining sterility is crucial for ensuring the safety of medications."

10.1 Can you identify an instance of non-sterile mixing activity?

a) Preparing a syringe for an injection

b) Making a powdered medication ready for use

c) Combining two oral liquid medications

d) Preparing a sterile IV solution

10.1 Answer: c) Combining two oral liquid medications

10.2 What is the role of laminar airflow hoods in sterile mixing?

a) To create a sterile environment for mixing

b) To regulate the temperature and humidity in the mixing area

c) To avoid cross-contamination between different drugs

d) To keep track of air quality during mixing processes

10.2 Answer: a) To create a sterile environment for mixing

10.3 Can you identify an instance of high-risk level mixing?

a) Preparing an oral suspension from commercially available tablets

b) Repackaging solid dosage forms into unit-dose containers

c) Mixing a sterile IV admixture for a patient

d) Mixing a topical cream with non-sterile ingredients

10.3 Answer: c) Mixing a sterile IV admixture for a patient

10.4 What is the correct way to put on sterile gloves when preparing a sterile compound?

a) The gloves should be put on after washing hands and sanitizing the gloves

b) The gloves should be put on with clean hands without washing them

c) The gloves should be put on using a sterile glove technique

d) Gloves are not required when mixing sterile preparations

10.4 Answer: c) The gloves should be put on using a sterile glove technique

10.5 What is the role of a laminar flow hood's prefilter?

a) To eliminate large particles from the air

b) To sterilize the air entering the hood

c) To maintain the temperature within the hood

d) To prevent contamination from the operator's hands

10.5 Answer: a) To eliminate large particles from the air

10.6 Can you identify an instance of an aseptic technique used in sterile mixing?

a) Wearing gloves throughout the entire mixing process

b) Using a fresh needle and syringe for each medication withdrawal

c) Using alcohol-based hand sanitizer instead of soap and water

d) Cleaning the work surface with a non-sterile cloth before mixing

10.6 Answer: b) Using a fresh needle and syringe for each medication withdrawal

10.7 Can you identify a critical site in sterile mixing?

a) The outer surface of an ampule

b) The top of a vial's rubber stopper

c) The exterior of a syringe barrel

d) The label on a medication bottle

10.7 Answer: b) The top of a vial's rubber stopper

10.8 What is the role of using a syringe filter in sterile mixing?

a) To eliminate particulate matter from the medication

b) To sterilize the medication before administration

c) To minimize the risk of contamination during mixing

d) To measure the precise volume of medication

10.8 Answer: a) To eliminate particulate matter from the medication

10.9 What does the term "Beyond-use Date" (BUD) mean in sterile mixing?

a) The date after which a mixed sterile preparation should not be used

b) The date on which a mixed sterile preparation was prepared

c) The date on which a mixed sterile preparation expires

d) The date after which a mixed sterile preparation can be used

10.9 Answer: a) The date after which a mixed sterile preparation should not be used

10.10 What should be done if a sterile mixing technician accidentally contaminates a sterile product?

a) The product should be thrown away, and the mixing process restarted

b) The product can be used if the contamination is minimal

c) The technician should continue mixing and complete the product

d) The product should be used only if it appears to be free of contamination

10.10 Answer: a) The product should be thrown away, and the mixing process restarted

Conclusion

As we wrap up this all-inclusive guide on gearing up for the Pharmacy Technician Certification Board Exam (PTCB), it's a moment to reflect, rejoice, and anticipate the thrilling prospects that await you. Throughout this process, you've demonstrated determination, tenacity, and a pursuit of excellence, traits that will be invaluable in your career as a certified pharmacy technician.

The multiple-choice questions (MCQs) have been a crucial part of your preparation, enabling you to evaluate your understanding and pinpoint your strong points and areas needing more focus. By tackling these questions, you've honed your critical thinking abilities and attained a profound comprehension of the crucial concepts and principles vital for your role as a pharmacy technician.

The sections in this guide have given you a thorough understanding of the PTCB exam, the duties and practice scope of a pharmacy technician, strategies for exam preparation, and tips for test-day tactics. You've also delved into the significance of pharmacy technicians in healthcare and the resources available for your ongoing professional development.

Now, as you ponder on your journey, take a moment to applaud your success. The time, effort, and dedication you've put into your preparation is a victory in itself. The knowledge and skills you've acquired throughout this process will lay the groundwork for a rewarding career in the pharmacy sector.

As you progress, bear in mind the significance of patient care, medication safety, and effective communication. Seize every chance to positively influence the lives of patients and champion their well-being. Your role as a certified pharmacy technician is vital to the healthcare system, and your pursuit of excellence will enhance the overall quality of patient care.

In this constantly changing field, it's crucial to keep advancing your professional growth and development. Look for opportunities for continuing education and stay abreast of the latest developments in pharmaceutical practices and technology. By staying informed and broadening your knowledge, you will establish yourself as a valuable resource in the pharmacy sector.

As you set off on your career, remember that success isn't solely gauged by passing an exam, but by the impact you make on patients' lives and the satisfaction you derive from your work. Welcome each challenge as a chance for growth and learning, and approach each day with enthusiasm, professionalism, and a commitment to delivering the highest standard of care.

Kudos on completing this PTCB Exam preparation journey. You've shown resilience, commitment, and a passion for your chosen field. As you step into the world of pharmacy, remember that your journey is just starting. The opportunities and rewards that lie ahead are boundless. Embrace them wholeheartedly and continue to aim for excellence in all you do.

Remember, you're part of a dynamic and essential profession that plays a pivotal role in healthcare. Your knowledge, skills, and dedication will positively affect the lives of numerous patients. Remain inquisitive, compassionate, and never cease learning. Your journey as a certified pharmacy technician has just started, and it promises a fulfilling and meaningful career.

Printed in Great Britain
by Amazon

33789483R00086